FINDING THE HIDDEN ALLERGEN

If someone in your family is allergic to corn, you probably are very careful to avoid serving cornflakes, popcorn, succotash and tortilla chips, but do you know that you should also avoid foods that contain caramel color, Vitamin C, sorbitol, vinegar, or baking powder—food additives that are often derived from corn or may contain cornstarch? And in the supermarket, would you be able to choose wisely between Homestyle *Ragu* Spaghetti Sauce and *Ragu*'s Marinara Sauce, correctly avoiding the one that contains corn syrup?

This is the kind of essential—sometimes life-saving—information you will learn in—

THE ALLERGY GUIDE TO BRAND-NAME FOODS AND FOOD ADDITIVES

STEPHANIE BERNARDO JOHNS is a researcher and writer who specializes in health and medical topics. She lives in New Jersey and has a son with a serious allergy to nuts. Her previous books are *The Ultimate Checklist* and *The Ethnic Almanac*.

THE ALLERGY GUIDE TO BRAND-NAME FOODS AND FOOD ADDITIVES

by

Stephanie Bernardo Johns

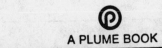

A PLUME BOOK

NEW AMERICAN LIBRARY

NEW YORK AND SCARBOROUGH, ONTARIO

PUBLISHER'S NOTE

The ideas, procedures, and suggestions contained in this book are not intended as a substitute for consulting with your physician. All matters regarding your health require medical supervision.

NAL BOOKS ARE AVAILABLE AT QUANTITY DISCOUNTS WHEN USED TO PROMOTE PRODUCTS OR SERVICES. FOR INFORMATION PLEASE WRITE TO PREMIUM MARKETING DIVISION. NEW AMERICAN LIBRARY. 1633 BROADWAY. NEW YORK. NEW YORK 10019.

PLUME TRADEMARK REG. U.S. PAT. OFF. AND FOREIGN COUNTRIES
REGISTERED TRADEMARK—MARCA REGISTRADA
HECHO EN BRATTLEBORO, VT., U.S.A.

SIGNET, SIGNET CLASSIC, MENTOR, ONYX, PLUME, MERIDIAN and NAL BOOKS are published *in the United States* by NAL PENGUIN INC., 1633 Broadway, New York, New York 10019, *in Canada* by The New American Library of Canada Limited, 81 Mack Avenue, Scarborough, Ontario M1L 1M8

Library of Congress Cataloging-in-Publication Data

Johns, Stephanie Bernardo.
  The allergy guide to brand-name foods and food additives / by Stephanie Bernardo Johns.
    p.   cm.
  ISBN 0-452-26059-0
  1. Food allergy—Popular works. 2. Food—Analysis. I. Title.
RC596.J64   1988   87-34017
616.9′ 75—dc19   CIP

First Printing, May, 1988
1 2 3 4 5 6 7 8 9
PRINTED IN THE UNITED STATES OF AMERICA

For David—so you'll never be caught off guard again
by chocolate-covered cherries with marzipan
or doughnuts laced with filbert nuts
and
For Christopher—so I'll always remember to check
the ice cream label for eggs.

Love,
Mom

Contents

ACKNOWLEDGMENTS

There are almost 4,000—a not inconsiderable number—listings in this edition but I hope many more manufacturers and fast-food chains will cooperate in the future to provide a more complete reference guide for all those consumers who have to ask, "Does it have milk?" or "Does it contain peanuts?" before they dare take a bite.

For their assistance with this volume, I'd like to thank Priscilla Harcourt, who spent many long hours at McGill University poring over medical journals, and Stephen and Emily Rizzo, who spent countless hours caring for Christopher so this book could be written. I'd also like to thank Michael for his patience and support, and the hundreds of manufacturers, researchers, physicians, and company representatives who supplied much of the information that appears in this book:

(Donna R. Tainter) Alberto Culver Co.; (Barbara McCabe) Allied Old English, Inc.; (Lani Benjamin) Anderson Bakery Co., Inc.; Anglo-Dietetics, Ltd.; (Richard La Calamito) American Bakeries Co.; Arby's; (Mary Webber) Armour Food Company; (Carol Davis) Armour Frozen Food; (Michelle Fiorillo) Arnold & Co., Inc.; (Boyd M. Foster) Arrowhead Mills, Inc.; (Charlotte Perry) The Great Atlantic & Pacific Tea Co., Inc.;

(Kaye Lambros) Bachman Co.; (Millie Roberson) Bartles & James Co.; (Lisa D. Caheen) Baskin-Robbins; (T. N. Trinchese) Beatrice Hunt/Wesson; (Richard C. Theur) Beech-Nut Nutrition Corp.; (Beth Miller) Beecham Products; (David Barash) Ben & Jerry's; (Myra Kaye) Bernard Food Industries, Inc.; Best Foods; (Lou E. Hauptman) R. C. Bigelow, Inc.; (Janet K. Werner) Bil-Mar Foods, Inc.; (Donna A. Giammakis) Bongrain International; (Janet Davis) Borden, Inc.; (Penelope Edwards) Bronson Pharmaceuticals; (June Scott) Burger King Corp.;

Cadbury Schweppes, Ltd.; (Jacquelin Marsh) Campbell Taggart, Inc.; (Helen McLean) Cantisano Foods, Inc.; (L. E. Abramson) Carnation; (Rhonda Jones) Celestial Seasonings; (Raleigh J. Shook) Charles Chips; (Terry Contos) Charms Co.; (Anita Johnson) Chef Francisco, Inc.; Dr. William Jay Chernack, Morristown, N.J.; Chico-San; (Walter Taylor) Chock Full O' Nuts; (Eileen M. Hamall) Church & Dwight Co., Inc.; (Louisa R. Kates) Church's Fried Chicken; (Thomas L. Ruble) Claussen Pickle Co.; Coca-Cola Foods; (Bob Burke) Columbo, Inc.; (Jean Tobey) Con Agra Consumer Frozen Food Companies; Concord Foods, Inc.; (Dr. David F. Owen) Continental Baking Co.; (Christine Pines) CPC International, Inc.; (Gail L. Becker) Cumberland Packing Corp.; Dr. Mary Custer, Food & Drug Administration;

(Susan J. Tomassetti) Dairymen, Inc.; (Dorothy R. Young) The Dannon Co., Inc.; DeBoles Nutritional Foods, Inc.; Del Monte Corp.; (Steven C. Klein) Denk Baking Corp.; (Janice Scandella) Dole Processed Foods Co.; Duffy-Mott Co., Inc.;

(Lois A. Heur) Eagle Snacks, Inc.; (Randy Feldman) Edward & Sons Trading Co.; (Sam M. Wylde, Jr.) Ener-G-Foods, Inc.; (Linda Peace) Entenmann's, Inc.; (Phyllis Rosenthal) Equal/Nutrasweet Products, Inc.; (Lynn C. Rajewski) Erewhon, Inc.; Delegation of the Commission of the European Communities;

(Katie Ross) Famous Amos Chocolate Chip Cookie Co.; (Gail Hartman) Fantastic Foods, Inc.; (Louis P. Richard) Fearn Natural Foods; (Rosalind Rota) Ferrara Foods and Confections, Inc.; Dr. Mary Ruth Fox; R. T. French Co.; (Hillary S. Brodsky) Fromageries Bel, Inc.; (Pat Hug) Frozfruit;

(Dr. Gene Grossman) General Foods; General Mills; Gerber Products Co.; (Mindy D. Goldenberg) Goldenberg Candy Co.; (Carol V. DeVito) Goodman Egg Noodle Products; (Faye Brophy) The Gorton Group; W. R. Grace & Co.; Grandma's Molasses; Gravymaster, Inc.;

Häagen-Dazs Ice Cream; Hanover Brands; L. S. Heath & Sons, Inc.; (Frances X. Beiles) Henry Heide, Inc.; (George Mateljan) Health Valley Foods; (John C. Long, Lael M. Moynihan) Hershey Foods Corp.; (Kay Hoffman) Hillshire Farm Co.; (Jerry Heflin) Hollywood Brands, Inc.; (Dale Arett) Hormel;

(Virginia Martin) Interbake Foods, Inc.; (Diane Wieland) International Multifoods; Iroquois Grocery Products;

(Charles T. Wegner III) Jel Sert Co.; (Frances Jones) Jones Dairy Farm; (William F. Sommers) Just Born, Inc.;

Kellogg's; (Elaine T. Beatson) Kikkoman International Inc.; Knott's Berry Farm; Kraft, Inc. Dairy Group; (Cynthia Raabe Hussong) Kroger Co.;

(Martha M. Turkington) Lactaid, Inc.; Land O' Lakes, Inc.; (Murray Lender) Lender's Bagel Bakery, Inc.; (George Schrenzel) Life Tone Int., Inc.; (Marie McDermott) Thomas J. Lipton, Inc.; Louis Rich; (N.A. Ruppert) Luden's, Inc.;

(Ruthy Mottram) M&M/Mars; Manischewitz; (Mary F. Maguire) Marriott Corp.; (Chrisopher Garrity) McDonald's Corp.; McCormick & Co., Inc.; Dr. Dean D. Metcalfe, National Institutes of Health; Mrs. Paul's Kitchens; (Nancy Williams) Mrs. Smith's Frozen Foods Co.; Myers;

(Caroline Fee) Nabisco Brands, Inc.; (Paula J. Kalajian) Near East Food Products, Inc.; (Carol Epstein) Nestlé Foods Corp.; Nissin Foods (USA) Co., Inc.; (Peter L. Dray) Nutrition Industries Corp.;

(Elizabeth A. Nichols) Ocean Spray Cranberries, Inc.; Ogden Food Products Corp.; Victoria L. Olejer, University of Texas, San Antonio; (Merine Heberger) Ore-Ida Foods, Inc.; Organic Milling Co., Inc.; The Original Philadelphia Pretzel; (Jean Cowden) Oscar Mayer Foods Corp.;

(B. W. Crosby) Pepperidge Farm, Inc.; (Anita Pancotto, Mary Perpich) Pepsi-Cola USA; (Janet L. Turnbough) Pet, Inc.; (Pat Godfrey) Pillsbury Co.; (Brenda Dellolio) Popsicle, Inc.; Pollio Dairy Products Corp.; (J. Edward Hunter) Procter & Gamble; (Fran Hill) Progresso Quality Foods;

(P. Nancy Mastey) Quaker Maid Meats; (Eileen Lochhead) Quaker Oats Co.;

(Linda Perham) Ragu Foods, Inc.; (Pat Klingler) Ralston Purina Co.; (Mike Trivedi) Red Cheek; (Dawn A. Wolf) Rich Products Corp.; (Peter R. Floersheimer) Ritter Food; (Robbie Mayberry) Riviana Foods, Inc.; (Greg C. Johnson) Russell Stover Candies;

(Lori A. Miller) SCM Corp.; Salada Foods, Inc.; (Sue Neros) Sandoz Nutrition; (Peg Ransom) Kitchens of Sara Lee; (Lea Frey) Shaffer, Clarke & Co., Inc.; (Lucille Canfara) Shasta Beverages, Inc.; J. M. Smucker Co.; (Rhonda Peek) Snack Master; Snapple Juice Co.; Speas Farm Co.; (Helen Andersen) Specialty Brands, Inc.; Stouffer Foods Corp.; Sun Diamond Growers of California; (Carol M. Gogg) Sunshine Biscuits, Inc.; (Thomas J. Wolfe) Switzer Clark;

(Louis P. Neeb) Taco Villa, Inc.; Dr. Stephen L. Taylor, Food Research Institute, University of Wisconsin; (Eileen Frech) S. B. Thomas, Inc.; (Lori E. Gurley) Tropicana Products, Inc.; (Jay Benham) Tyson Foods, Inc.;

Uncle Ben's, Inc.; (Timothy F. Twardzik) Uteeco, Inc.; (Debra M. Snyder) Utz Quality Foods, Inc.;

Ventre Packing Co., Inc.; Venus Wafers, Inc.; (Justine R. Good) Vlasic Foods, Inc.;

(Paul Berks) Walden Farms; (Lucinda Kaufman) Walnut Acres; Welch Foods, Inc.; Wendy's International Inc.; Willie Wonka Brands; Wilton Enterprises; (Gillian Wood) Worthington Foods, Inc.;

Y & S Candies; (Dr. John Yunginger) Mayo Clinic, Rochester, Minnesota.

THE ALLERGY GUIDE TO BRAND-NAME FOODS AND FOOD ADDITIVES

Introduction:
Allergies and
Brand-Name Foods

"One man's meat . . ."

Food *allergy* is a general term used to describe any adverse reaction connected with the ingestion of certain foods or food ingedients. These reactions are usually caused by a breakdown in the body's immune system, causing it to attack ordinarily harmless substances such as food or food additives. Individual reactions to food allergies can be mild or severe, ranging from a runny nose, rashes, eczema, hives, and headaches to gastrointestinal upset, swelling, wheezing, asthma and, in rare cases, death.

Although milk, eggs, corn, soy, nuts, peanuts, and wheat are among the most common offenders, in truth, *any* food or food additive can cause an allergic response. As Dr. Dean D. Metcalfe, Senior Clinical Investigator at the National Institutes of Health, once remarked: "Having had [as a patient] one lady who had a systemic life-threatening reaction to carrots, I no longer accept any antigen as impossible to cause a life-threatening reaction."

How Common Are Food Allergies?

The Asthma and Allergy Foundation (AAF) estimates that 35 million Americans, or about 17 percent of the population, suffer from significant allergies. Of that number, the AAF estimates at least 3 million Americans are allergic to food. But the U.S. Department of Agriculture believes that figure is even higher, claiming that some *34 million* adults and children are "allergic to some food ingredients."

Although it may not be clear exactly how many Americans suffer from food allergies, what is clear is that the subject is perceived to be a problem by a significant number of consumers. In a recent survey of 200 women in 20 metropolitan areas, conducted by the Consumer Research Department of *Good Housekeeping* magazine, 30 percent of the women polled (or a member of their families) were allergic to some food products. And 22 percent stated that they regularly avoided certain foods or food additives in their families' diets.

A Life-Threatening Situation

For many Americans, avoiding food allergens is not a matter of convenience, but a matter of life and death. Those who suffer from immediate reactions to foods such as nuts, peanuts, eggs, and shellfish, can, on rare occasions, experience dangerous reactions such as anaphylactic shock or rapid swelling of the throat and upper windpipe that can lead to suffocation.

My son, David, is violently allergic to nuts. At the first bite of a nut-laced food he can feel his throat start to swell and itch. If he *swallows* that food, he knows nausea and vomiting will result, as well as hives, swelling, and nasal congestion. Because of his allergy he carefully avoids fruitcakes, nut-laced cookies, granola, rocky road ice cream, and almond-flavored sweets. But there have been times when he was caught off guard by such seemingly innocent foods as chocolate-covered cherries (which are sometimes surrounded with marzipan), and certain brands of cakes and pastries, such as Entenmann's Country Style Donuts, which include ground filbert nuts. Because his allergy is so severe, David is always careful to read the labels of packaged foods; and if he is uncertain of a main course or a dessert being served at a restaurant or a friend's home, he politely declines, reasoning that it is better to be "safe and hungry" than to take a chance.

Tragically, there are allergic individuals who *die* each year because they were misinformed about the ingredients and wrongly assumed a food was safe to eat, or because they underestimated the severity of their food sensitivity. At a recent meeting of the

Food and Drug Administration's Ad Hoc Advisory Committee on Hypersensitivity to Food Constituents, a woman from Salimar, Florida, whose daughter had died in 1986 after eating two small cookies that contained ground peanuts, testified: "We never even heard the words 'anaphylaxis' or 'anaphylactic shock.' . . . We were never given even a clue that this [allergy] could be life-threatening. . . . Had we even an inkling of the gravity of the situation, we could have been a bit more prepared and possibly could have saved her life. . . ."

Fortunately, most individuals who suffer from food allergies will never run the risk of death following dietary indiscretion. At the worst, they will subject themselves to bouts of nausea and vomiting, or they will develop hives, headaches, abdominal pain, or other milder symptoms, such as canker sores, rashes, irritability, or mood swings.

Yet with so many choices of prepared food available in the marketplace, there's no reason why a food-sensitive consumer should ever suffer *any* distress—*if* he or she chooses brands wisely and is careful to avoid any and all substances that might contain allergenic ingredients.

Homemade Is Still Best

Many popular books on the subject of food allergy contain recipes for wheat-free, egg-free, or corn-free cakes, cookies, and pies, which are also free of unnecessary chemicals and additives. Compare a cookbook recipe for white bread to the label of a supermarket brand—the homemade recipe may call for flour, butter, sugar, yeast, and salt; there aren't any "extras" such as corn syrup, mono- and diglycerides, whey solids, calcium propionate, or artificial colors. Without a doubt, homemade food is superior in taste and quality to most store-bought products. But because man does not live by home-baked bread alone, and because there are times when only a Big Mac or a Creamsicle will do, it is especially important for a food-sensitive consumer to choose snacks wisely. It doesn't make sense for a peanut-sensitive consumer to buy French fries cooked in peanut oil or a chocolate bar containing emulsifiers that may have been derived from peanuts when there are dozens of safer choices in the marketplace.

The Aims of This Book

When you first embark on a special diet designed to eliminate corn, eggs, milk, nuts, soybeans, peanuts, wheat, or any other food, it can be quite time-consuming to stand in the supermarket aisles, reading labels as you shop. But eventually, when you discover which manufacturers routinely use peanut oil or corn oil to fry foods, and which use cottonseed oil or soybean oil in their baked goods, you learn which brands of cookies or potato chips you can safely eat and which brands should be avoided.

This book was written to help take some of the mystery out of processed foods and food additives, making it easier for the food-sensitive reader to stick to a particular diet. It was also written to save you the trouble of writing to several hundred manufacturers to request information about their food products.

This book can be an invaluable tool for anyone who wants to avoid corn, eggs, milk, nuts, peanuts, soy, wheat, or any by-products or additives that are derived from these seven substances. However, this book is not intended as medical advice—it is merely a guide to help food-sensitive individuals make wise, informed decisions about the food they buy and eat.

Buying and Preparing Allergen-Free Food

Friends who are allergic to milk have been advised by their physicians to avoid not only dairy products, but *all* foods that contain whey, caseinate, and other milk by-products that are common ingredients in salad dressings, baked goods, and frozen foods. Similarly, most dieticians and allergists advise their patients, especially those who are on elimination diets, to determine which foods they are allergic to, to avoid *all forms* of corn, eggs, wheat, soy, or whatever foods seem to cause them problems.

If someone in your family were allergic to corn or was trying to avoid corn in his diet, you would probably be careful to avoid serving him cornflakes, popcorn, succotash, and tortilla chips, but would you also avoid foods that contain caramel color, vitamin C, sorbitol, vinegar, or baking powder—food additives that are often derived from corn or may contain cornstarch? And in the supermarket, would you be able to choose wisely between

Homestyle Ragu spaghetti sauce and Ragu's Marinara Sauce, correctly avoiding the one that contains corn syrup?

Too often, a physician or allergist will send a patient home with vague instructions to "Avoid corn and all products made from corn." The physician might provide a partial list of obvious food ingredients made from corn, such as corn syrup and hominy grits, but what about all those food additives? Does a candy bar with lecithin contain "corn"? How about a frozen pizza with sodium erythrobate?

Of course, most popular allergy books advise food-sensitive readers to avoid *all* processed foods and foods with additives, preservatives, and other chemical ingredients. That's good advice for anyone, but in our fast-paced world it is often impossible to avoid eating *some* processed food, especially when traveling or eating in a restaurant. So for those times when you must choose between the "lesser of two evils," wouldn't it be comforting to know which brands of cake or cookies contained milk, nuts, or corn sweeteners? And whether it was better to order a box of Chicken McNuggets or a Burger King Whopper for lunch?

Always Read the Fine Print

When Coca-Cola introduced the "new" Coke several years ago, there was endless press coverage and discussion about which formula was better—the old, "Classic" Coke, or the new, "improved" version. Although Coke's formula is a secret, most soft-drink connoisseurs contend that the difference in taste between the original Coke and the New Coke was due to the shift from sugar to high fructose corn syrup as a sweetener.

Before the old version was reintroduced, loyal Coca-Cola fans who disliked the new formula were importing their Coke from Canada, where sugar, not corn syrup, is still king. And on a recent visit to Montreal I was surprised to find that not only Coke, but many other familiar brand-name products have slightly different ingredients North of the border. So before you drink a bottle of soda pop or eat a bag of potato chips in a foreign country, check the label—the name may be the same, but the product formulation may be slightly different to accommodate regional tastes.

The Name of the Game Is Substitution

Every day, dozens of companies change their recipes for brand-name foods without attracting any attention whatsoever from the press or the public. Almost every product that you ate as a child has probably had subtle changes made in its basic recipe in response to the changing market price of vegetable oils, sweeteners, and other ingredients. A baker might substitute almonds for hazelnuts in a coffee-cake topping, or a snack manufacturer might fry one batch of potato chips in cottonseed oil and the next in soybean oil. In fact, so much shifting—from soybean oil to cottonseed, or from corn flour to wheat flour—is done these days that many labels carry a list of alternatives to accommodate recipe changes for some cost-sensitive ingredients. Many national fast-food chains that rely on regional suppliers for breads, salad dressings, and milk-shake mixes are unable to provide exact ingredient information because their food products may vary from one state to the next. Most of these changes have little effect on the ultimate taste of the product, and little effect on the nutrition or health of the consumer, *except* if the consumer happens to be allergic to any of the new ingredients.

Because the proprietary formulas for artificial flavors and colors could not be determined, this book made no provision for such ingredients. Most manufacturers assert that these chemicals are either synthetically derived and thus free of any food proteins that could cause allergy, or else they are used in such miniscule amounts that even the most highly sensitive individual would not be bothered by any of the original food products. If you believe that food colors or flavors might be a problem, however, avoidance is the best course of action.

Every attempt was made to ensure that the data in this book were accurate, but because of the possibility of formula changes or typographical errors, the label is always the ultimate source of information.

Methods of Research

The idea for this book began more than 12 years ago when my son, David, became ill after eating a chocolate-covered cherry. I knew he was allergic to nuts, but until I wrote to that candy manufacturer I never knew that chocolate-covered cherries could contain marzipan (almond paste).

By reading every label and carefully avoiding any unlabeled foods that might contain nuts, several years passed before David had another adverse reaction. This time it was not ignorance, but complacency that caused the problem. An innocent-looking dough-nut, offered by a friend, was accepted. Neither of us thought to ask if it contained nuts, because we never imagined that a plain pastry, without a crumb topping, could contain ground filbert nuts.

When David felt his throat start to close after the first bite of doughnut, we knew that we couldn't afford ever to let our guard down again. That experience taught us to avoid certain brands of crumb cake, apple pie, and Danish pastry that list ground nuts on the ingredient label, yet look "harmless."

When I discovered there were dozens of innocent-looking foods with surprise ingredients (who would suspect pecans in barbecue sauce—Hunt's Thick & Rich, New Orleans style—or peanuts in plain M&M's or in Raisinets?), I realized many food-sensitive consumers could benefit from an allergy guide to brand-name foods.

To compile the data for this book I began, as any consumer might, by looking to product labels for information and manufac-turers' addresses. I sent almost 700 inquiries to national and regional manufacturers, yet fewer than half of those companies responded. Many letters were returned because the addresses listed on the product labels were insufficient for mailing; other letters were returned because the companies had relocated and left no forwarding addresses. Other companies responded by sending the wrong information (lists of calories, carbohydrates, or nutritional analyses), but the most shocking responses came from those companies that claimed not to have any information about the food they manufacture.

Some large corporations, perhaps out of fear of lawsuits, claimed they could not flatly state that any food they manufactured was free of, say, corn or wheat, because of the incidental additives that might be present and are not required by law to be listed on the label. (Examples of incidental additives or ingredients in-clude: fats used to grease baking pans; butter or vegetable oils or corn meal used as a carrier for beta-carotene or other colors; or yeast-nutrients, which might accompany the yeast added to bread or cake batter.) Although these additives are present in extremely minute, or trace quantities, and have never been proven to be a problem to even the most exquisitely sensitive consumer, the fact remains that most food manufacturers don't ask their suppliers of yeast or coloring about the exact additives, hence they have no way of knowing if corn, wheat, soy, or other allergens are present.

A few manufacturers said they preferred to answer individual requests from consumers on specific allergens such as corn, milk, or wheat. But many hedged when asked about even the simplest ingredients. One pickle manufacturer admitted that the vinegar used in his products might be corn-based or wheat-based—he didn't know and didn't want to be on record stating that his pickles contained corn or wheat, preferring to let consumers form their own opinions from the facts on the label. (I confronted that problem by listing both allergens as possibilities whenever a manufacturer was unclear about his ingredient sources.)

Only two large manufacturers refused to cooperate because they feared that a book, even one that was updated annually, could be inaccurate when product formulations changed. However, any consumer who routinely buys a brand-name product would be at the same disadvantage if he didn't read the label every time he made a new purchase, because no book, nor any corporate brochure can ever take the place of the ingredient statement. To illustrate this point: Several weeks ago I noticed that a package of Stella D'Oro cookies (Lady Stella Assortment) that I had bought, listed walnuts as an ingredient. My son didn't eat any of those cookies, but he has in the past, and I don't remember seeing walnuts listed on the ingredient label before. Because it is an "assortment" of cookies, the simplest explanation is that the assortment changes from one week to the next, and although walnuts were not apparent in any cookies in this particular package, they might be in the next package. And once again I learned the importance of reading the label, because you can't always tell a book, or a cookie, by its cover.

A Few Words
About Food Additives

How many times have you bitten into a favorite childhood food such as a marshmallow pie, a frozen fudge bar, or a piece of candy, only to remark, "It doesn't taste as good as it did when I was a kid"? In the "old days"—before the introduction of space-age emulsifiers, stabilizers, chemical preservatives, and antioxidants, and prior to the current glut of prepared, frozen, microwaveable meals and snacks—food *was* simpler. The baker on the corner didn't use emulsifiers such as sodium stearoyl lactylate to prevent the separation of water and fat, nor did he use carob bean gum or xanthan gum to thicken the fillings in his Danish pastries; your soft drinks, for the most part, were formulated completely with sugar; and the abbreviation BHA and BHT were rarely found in the fine print on cereal boxes. So the taste that you remembered as a child *was* different, because food manufacturing has changed.

Food additives have been playing an ever-increasing role in American food production as consumers spend more and more of their food dollars on processed, prepared, and convenience items. But despite the addition of hundreds of multisyllabic chemicals and preservatives of dubious nutritional value, not all of the changes in food production have been for the worse. Cookies that used to be baked with lard now contain vegetable shortening in deference to the public's new enlightened consciousness about cholesterol. And many more health-conscious meals and snacks are generally available, in both health-food stores and supermarkets.

What Is a Food Additive?

Under the Food, Drug and Cosmetic Act a "food additive" is any substance that directly or indirectly becomes a component of a food product or otherwise affects the characteristics of that food. The most widely used food additives are salt, sugar, and corn syrup, but any substance that is used to produce, process, treat, package, preserve, transport, or store food is considered an "additive."

Direct additives are those ingredients that are part of the recipe; they are added *directly* to foods and their presence must be indicated on the label. Indirect additives are substances that are not added to the food per se, but may be present in very small amounts as a result of some phase of production, processing, storage, or packaging.

When Is a Food Additive Not an Ingredient?

There are more than 2,800 direct food additives and as many as 10,000 indirect additives that can become incorporated in various foods during processing, packaging, and storage. The most predominant additives are sugar, salt, and corn syrup; these plus citric acid, baking soda, vegetable colors, mustard, and pepper account for more than 98 percent (by weight) of all food additives used in the United States.

All ingredients and *direct additives* must be listed on the product label in descending order according to weight. Although all additives must be approved for safety by the Food and Drug Administration (FDA) and the Food Safety and Inspection Service (FSIS) of the U.S. Department of Agriculture (USDA), the law does not require *indirect additives* to appear on the ingredient label.

Some indirect or incidental additives result as a side reaction in the manufacturing process. For example, in the manufacture of corn syrup, hydrochloric acid (HCl) is used to accelerate the reaction, and sodium hydroxide (NaOH) is used to neutralize the hydrochloric acid. The combination of HCl and NaOH may produce a tiny amount of salt (NaCl); however, because salt was not intended to be part of the finished food product, the law does not require it to be listed on the ingredient label.

Other indirect additives can also be added to foods from packaging materials. If, for example, a corn-based plastic wrapper were used to package Pasteurized Process American Cheese Food, it is possible that some corn protein, or other chemicals such as plasticizers, could migrate from the wrapper to the cheese.

In truth, it would be impossible for a manufacturer to guess at the number of incidental reactions that might occur when food is processed. Nor is there any evidence to suggest that such trace amounts of food protein or chemicals are grave health concerns for the majority of consumers. The fact that such incidental additives do exist, however, only serves to point out the complexity of trying to understand the how and why of food allergy.

There's More to an Additive than Meets the Eye

When I first conceived the idea for this book, I naively assumed it would be a fairly straightforward task to examine the labels of several thousand prepared foods and check which ones contained corn, egg, milk, nuts, peanuts, soy, and wheat—seven of the most common food allergens. What I neglected to consider before I began this project were the hundreds of food additives that have become part of the American chemical feast. Butylated hydroxyanisole (BHA), butylated hydroxytoluene (BHT) monosodium glutamate (MSG), calcium disodium EDTA, lecithin, mono- and diglycerides—all are fairly common words on most ingredient labels these days, yet I had no idea whether they had been derived from any food allergens. So my first task was to discover what substances common food additives are derived from, and then to find out if these additives could be considered a "problem" for someone on a wheat-free, corn-free, or soy-free diet.

In my search for answers I consulted dozens of texts on food processing, chemical technology, chemistry, government regulations, and medicine; I contacted dozens of manufacturers, allergists, and research scientists, and looked to the medical literature for the most current information on the subject of food additives and hypersensitivity. In the end, I came to the conclusion that food additives are a "gray" area: sensitive individuals have had reactions to additives such as MSG and tartrazine (FD&C No. 5);

however, scientific proof—in the form of controlled, double-blind experiments—is lacking to create a consensus on whether these substances are also a problem for the food sensitive.

Some physicians and food scientists contend that anytime a food such as corn or wheat is transformed into another substance such as alcohol, malt syrup, or monosodium glutamate, the allergenic properties of the original protein have been totally changed, hence these derivatives should not pose a problem for corn- or wheat-sensitive patients. Yet, some dieticians and allergists believe such additives can have an adverse effect on some patients' health, especially those who suffer from celiac disease, a food intolerance that demands total avoidance of gluten and products made from wheat, rye, buckwheat, and other gluten-containing grains. Recent research has shown that even though some celiacs may be able to tolerate small amounts of gluten in their daily diet without suffering bloating or diarrhea, the ingestion of gluten may have an adverse effect on their intestinal villi and place them at an increased risk for malignancy of the small intestine.

With "true" food allergies (those that are immunologic reactions to the ingestion of a food or food additive), total avoidance of all food products is also recommended. For example, if someone was allergic to peanuts and successfully avoided all peanut products for several years, theory holds that his IgE titers to peanut protein would decrease over time, making his reactions less severe. If this person is not totally successful in avoiding the protein to which he is sensitive, however, his IgE titers will remain at a high level, increasing the chances of a severe attack.

Also, despite the fact that several researchers have shown that seed oils, such as soybean or peanut, do not contain soy or peanut protein, nonetheless there are many patients who claim to have reactions to corn oil, peanut oil, and other such products.

Although much of the information obtained from patients is what scientists would call "anecdotal" (meaning there wasn't a physician on hand to perform a controlled experiment to prove that the additives in question were responsible for the allergic symptoms), and many physicians might question whether the symptoms were psychosomatic or caused by another antigen, still I felt that patients' experiences could not be ignored. After all, "what you don't eat, can't hurt you."

When an additive was derived from more than one food crop, I felt it was important to list all possible sources so food-allergic consumers would be aware that not all additives with the same name have the exact same chemical composition. Consider the case of *lecithin*, a common emulsifier that can be derived from corn, eggs, peanuts, or soybeans. Commercial lecithin products typically contain only about 15-percent *pure* lecithin (a phosphatide). These lecithins also contain about 30-percent fatty oil, and "with respect to minor constituents, there are differences between the commercial lecithins that are derived from different sources."* I don't know whether any of these "differences" include protein fractions that could cause an allergic reaction, nor could I find any scientific experiments to prove lecithin was a problem to food-sensitive patients, but in the absence of any scientific "proof" to the contrary, I took the cautious approach. Thus if a food contained lecithin, but the label did not qualify it as soya lecithin or vegetable lecithin, I did not presume to guess its origin and indicated that the product might contain corn, eggs, peanuts, and soy.

If you are sensitive to corn, yet have never experienced a problem after eating a candy bar with lecithin added, it could mean one of three things: that the lecithin was actually derived from soy, eggs, or peanuts; or the lecithin, even though derived from corn, did not contain any allergenic substances; or your allergies are not severe enough to be triggered by such trace amounts of protein.

Because there are individuals who are so sensitive they claim to react to even the smell of an offensive substance, I felt their needs could not be ignored. To make this book truly useful, I took the most conservative viewpoint and sided with those physicians who advise their patients to avoid *any and all forms* of a troublesome food.

---

*Kirk-Othmer Encyclopedia of Chemical Technology.

Food Additives and Possible Allergens

Food Additive or Ingredient	CORN	EGGS	MILK	NUTS	PEANUT	SOY	WHEAT
ALBUMEN		E					
ALBUMIN		E					
ALCOHOL	C						W
ALCOHOLIC BEVERAGES:							
Bourbon	C						W
Corn Whiskey	C						W
Gin	C						W
Holland Gin	C						W
Rye	C						W
Scotch	C						W
Vodka	C						W
Whiskey	C						W
ASCORBIC ACID	C						
BAKING POWDER	C						
BARLEY MALT							W
BETA-AMYLASE						S	
BETA-CAROTENE	C		M		P	S	
BROMINATED VEGETABLE OIL	C				P	S	
CALCIUM CITRATE	C					S	
CALCIUM LACTATE	C		M				
CALCIUM STEARATE	C				P	S	
CALCIUM STEAROYL-2-LACTYLATE	C		M		P	S	
CARAMEL COLOR	C		M				W
CASEIN			M				
CERELOSE	C						
CITRIC ACID	C						
CONALBUMEN		E					
CONFECTIONERS' SUGAR	C						
CORNSTARCH	C						
CORN SYRUP	C						
DEXTRIN	C						W
DEXTROSE	C						
DIGLYCERIDES	C				P	S	
DISODIUM GUANYLATE						S	
ERYTHORBIC ACID	C						
ESTER GUM	C				P	S	

Food Additive or Ingredient	CORN	EGGS	MILK	NUTS	PEANUT	SOY	WHEAT
ETHANOL	C						W
ETHYL ALCOHOL	C						W
FATTY ACIDS	C				P	S	
FATTY ALCOHOLS						S	
FLOUR							W
FOOD STARCH	C						W
FRUCTOSE	C						
FUMARIC ACID	C						
GLUCONIC ACID	C						
GLUCONO DELTA LACTONE	C						
GLUCOSE	C						
GLUTAMATES	C					S	W
GLUTEN							W
GLYCERIDES	C				P	S	
GLYCEROL	C				P	S	
GLYCERYL MONOSTEARATE	C		M		P	S	
HIGH FRUCTOSE CORN SYRUP	C						
HYDROGENATED VEGETABLE SHORTENING	C				P	S	
HYDROL	C						
HYDROLYZED VEGETABLE PROTEIN	C				P*	S	W
ISOMEROSE	C						
LACTALBUMIN			M				
LACTIC ACID	C		M				
LACTIC FERMENTING AGENTS			M				
LACTOSE			M				
LACTYLATED FATTY ACID ESTERS	C		M				
LECITHIN	C	E			P	S	
LEVULOSE	C						
LIPOXIDASE						S	
LIVETIN		E					
MALIC ACID	C						
MALT	C						W
MALT FLAVORING	C						W
MALT SYRUP	C						W
MALTED MILK			M				W
MALTODEXTRIN	C						W
MALTOL	C						W

Food Additive or Ingredient	CORN	EGGS	MILK	NUTS	PEANUT	SOY	WHEAT
MALTOSE	C					S	W
MANNITOL	C						
MISO						S	
MODIFIED CORNSTARCH	C						
MODIFIED FOOD STARCH	C						W
MODIFIED VEGETABLE PROTEIN	C				P*	S	W
MONOGLYCERIDE CITRATE	C					S	W
MSG/MONOSODIUM GLUTAMATE	C					S	W
MYRISTIC ACID			M				
NATTO						S	
OVALBUMIN		E					
OVOMUCIN		E					
OVOMUCOID		E					
PEPTONES		E	M			S	
POLYDEXTROSE	C						
POLYSORBATES	C				P	S	
POTASSIUM GLUCONATE	C						
PROPYLENE GLYCOL MONOSTEARATE	C				P	S	
SODIUM CITRATE	C						
SODIUM ERYTHROBATE	C						
SODIUM GLUCONATE	C						
SODIUM LACTATE	C		M				
SODIUM STEAROYL-2-LACTYLATE	C				P	S	
SORBASE						S	
SORBITANS	C				P	S	
SORBITOL	C						
SOY SAUCE						S	W
SOYA LECITHIN						S	
SOYA PROTEIN						S	
STARTER CULTURES			M				
STARTER DISTILLATE	C		M				
STEARIC ACID	C				P	S	
TEMPEH						S	
TOCOPHEROLS	C				P	S	
TOFU						S	
UREASE						S	
VANILLA EXTRACT	C						W
VEGETABLE OIL	C				P	S	

Food Additive or Ingredient	CORN	EGGS	MILK	NUTS	PEANUT	SOY	WHEAT
VINEGAR	C						W
VITAMIN C	C						
VITAMIN E						S	W
VITELLIN		E					
WHEY			M				
WHEY SOLIDS			M				
XANTHAN GUM	C						
ZEIN	C						

*Only in imported foods.

The Pleasures and Perils of Eating Out

The tragic death in 1986 of a Brown University coed who was allergic to peanuts and died after eating a bowl of chili that had been thickened with peanut butter only serves to remind us that danger lurks in every stew pot. The world of nouvelle cuisine is full of unexpected surprises; trendy restaurants may add goat cheese, tofu, peanut sauce, or walnut oil to salads, appetizers, or main courses.

To help you cope with the uncertainties of dining out, follow these suggestions for allergen-free meals:

• If the menu is written in a foreign language, or if it contains terms that you don't understand, *ask* for a translation. A friend once ordered *ris de veau* in a French restaurant, expecting a dish that contained rice and veal; what he got were sweetbreads. He isn't allergic to sweetbreads, just squeamish about eating thymus glands, but because it was a business lunch he couldn't afford to insult his hosts and had to savor every last morsel.

• If you are unsure of the contents of a dish—or if your allergies are life-threatening—ask the chef or the cook for a complete list of ingredients even if it seems unlikely that the dish could contain peanuts, nuts, or eggs.

• If you're invited to a friend's home, always offer to bring a casserole or a dessert that conforms to your special diet, so you won't be tempted by exotic unknowns.

• Always carry a snack when traveling. Some airlines will accommodate the dietary needs of passengers by providing special meals, but mistakes do happen. If you're sensitive to sulfites, you may not be able to eat *any* airline food; it may be best to tuck a piece of fruit or a homemade sandwich into your briefcase for emergencies.

• If you're allergic to nuts or peanuts, don't think that you can remove them from a prepared food and make it safe to eat. Even if you take the peanuts out of a bowl of mixed nuts, or remove the almonds from a green bean amandine casserole, some invisible traces of protein will still remain.

• Never eat a suspect food on an empty stomach. Food is absorbed at varying rates, depending upon the stomach's contents. If you have an anaphylactic reaction and your stomach has to be lavaged, the chances of removing the antigen are better if it has been consumed toward the end of the meal.

• Be careful of serving utensils; they can easily contaminate a safe food; cross-contamination can occur when food adheres to a spoon or knife. Be cautious at salad bars and buffets, where eggs, cheese, nuts, or corn can be transferred from one dish to another through a misplaced utensil. In one reported case, a peanut-sensitive individual became ill after eating a plain doughnut that had been in the same box as those with a peanut topping. The source of contamination was the waxed paper the clerk in the bakery used when he picked out the doughnuts: He grabbed the peanut doughnuts first, and subsequently transferred some peanut antigen to the plain doughnuts.

• Write to restaurant chains for information. Some chains, such as McDonald's and Burger King, have been responsive to the needs of the food-sensitive and have published booklets listing full ingredients for all of their products. Other chains, especially those that have built their reputation on secret recipes for chicken or fish, refuse to divulge their formulas. Despite the fact that Kentucky Fried Chicken has some 6,400 outlets worldwide and Americans eat about a third of a billion pounds of "finger-lickin' good" chicken each year, the company's nutritional brochure is vague ("Only the highest quality ingredients such as natural herbs and spices, flour, fresh buttermilk, carrots, and cabbage are used in KFC products") and of little use to those who suffer from food allergies and need to know if the Colonel uses corn, eggs, milk, wheat, soybean, or peanut oil in his batter. If more voices are heard clamoring for ingredient listings, the corporate officers will respond. Until then remember you, as the consumer, are in the driver's seat, and you can choose to take your business to those restaurants that are willing to divulge their ingredients.

How to Use This Book

The Allergy Guide to Brand-Name Foods and Food Additives can save you time and money by allowing you to do some "armchair shopping" before you visit the supermarket. That way, you don't have to stand in the aisles and read *every* label, and you don't run the risk of buying food that you'll have to discard. By using this book properly, you can limit your choice of potato chips or cookies to two to three "safe" brands and then double-check the product labels in the store to make sure they are safe for you to eat.

The alphabetical listings that begin on page 27 reflect the most recent data available on brand-name foods and fast-foods. Because manufacturers sometimes do change their recipes, however, the label is the ultimate source of information. Also, because incidental additives may have been included in some food products, be advised that this book does not endorse any foods as corn-free, wheat-free, egg-free, and so on. It is intended solely as a guide to help food-sensitive consumers make wise decisions about the food they buy.

Interpreting the Listings:

CORN—Most of the foods marked with a "C" contain corn, corn syrup, corn oil, or corn-derived additives such as caramel color, citric acid, vitamin C, xanthan gum, lecithin, modified food starch, malto-dextrin, and more. If you are extremely sensitive to corn-based products, beware: You might not be able to lick postage stamps or use plastic wrap. Corn is *everywhere*.

EGG—Most of the foods that rated an "E" contained eggs, egg whites, egg yolks, or lecithin, a food additive that can be derived from eggs.

MILK—The foods that are listed as containing milk were either made with milk, cream, buttermilk, butter, butterfat, yogurt, or cheese; or else they contained caramel color, lactic acid, calcium lactate, and other additives that may have been derived from milk or milk sugar. (Please note: Foods that have been marked with "M" in this book may still be "kosher," or "pareve." Jewish dietary law was not consulted with regard to additives such as lactic acid or calcium lactate, and under such laws these additives may not be considered to be milk-containing substances.)

NUTS—Coconuts and peanuts were *not* included in this listing because most researchers consider them to be different from "tree nuts," such as walnuts, almonds, and pecans. Other true nuts include pine nuts, Brazil nuts, shea nuts (an oil source), chestnuts, filberts (hazelnuts), and cashews.

PEANUTS—Foods that received a check in the peanut column most frequently contained peanut butter, ground peanuts, peanut oil; lecithin, mono- and diglycerides, ester gum, stearates, and other additives that may have been derived from peanut fat. Also, any imported foods that contain hydrolyzed vegetable protein (HVP) were marked with a "P," because European manufacturers sometimes use peanuts in the manufacture of HVP.

SOY—Foods marked with an "S" contain soybeans, soybean oil, tofu, miso, soy sauce, or texturized vegetable protein, as well as by-products of soybean processing such as glycerine, enzymes and tocopherols, and other fat-based additives that may have been derived from soy.

WHEAT/GLUTEN—All grains such as rye, oats, barley, buckwheat, and wheat are sources of gluten that should be avoided by those with a gluten intolerance; thus, it is possible for a "wheat-free" food to be marked with a "W" on the following list. Other products derived from wheat include starch, MSG (monosodium glutamate), malt, malt syrup, and malted milk.

NOTE: A check in any of the seven columns does not mean that a food definitely contains corn, egg, milk, nuts, peanut, wheat, or soy as an ingredient; it only means that it *might* contain that substance. Whenever there was a question about an ingredient all possible sources were indicated.

Because some manufacturers supplied ingredient lists, whereas others supplied information only on the allergens contained in their foods, it is conceivable that two food products with the same ingredients could have checks in different columns. Whenever a manufacturer stated that his products were, for example, corn-free, or wheat-free, I accepted his word that no corn or wheat protein was present. When I was forced to interpret the ingredient label, however, I had to take the most conservative approach possible and note all potential sources of an ingredient.

When In Doubt, Contact the Manufacturer

Many companies are highly responsive to the needs of consumers. Recently, when four consumers suffered allergic reactions to Hershey's Cocoa Creme Flavored New Trail Chocolate Covered Granola Bars, the company recalled 2.8 million granola bars when it was discovered that peanuts had mistakenly been added to the recipe.

Although none of these consumers could have anticipated that peanuts would be added by mistake, contamination is *always* a possibility when you buy prepared foods. A classic example cited by Dr. Stephen Taylor is the case of a peanut-sensitive individual who experienced a reaction to almond butter, which is made from pulverized almonds and is not supposed to contain peanuts or peanut butter. When Dr. Taylor inspected the plant where the almond butter was processed, he learned that the same production line had been used to make peanut butter. And as a result of incomplete cleaning of one small pipe, the first few jars of almond butter that came off the assembly line were contaminated with as much as 10-percent peanut protein.

Several months ago a friend who is allergic to nuts had an

immediate adverse reaction to Twining's Earl Grey Tea. He became short of breath, began to wheeze, and felt as if someone was squeezing his chest. A call to the manufacturer eased his mind—the flavoring used in the tea, bergamot oil, had been squeezed from a pear-shaped fruit, *Citrus bergamia*, that is grown on the island of Sicily, and did not contain any nut oils or essences. He was lucky. After several hours, and several doses of medication, his symptoms subsided, but if he had not been able to speak to someone about the ingredients, his fear might have compounded his symptoms. Anxiety over a food allergy can often cause a patient to hyperventilate if he believes he is in a life-threatening situation, and this "hyperventilation syndrome" can confuse the whole issue of food allergy, because the syndrome doesn't respond to normal medical treatment.

If you have a question about a food product, contact the manufacturer. Companies such as Nabisco, Oscar Mayer, Hormel, Best Foods, Burger King, McDonald's, and Stouffer's publish fact sheets to assist the special dietary needs of their consumers. Some small specialty companies, such as Ener-G, are even able to list all of the possible allergens from incidental additives used in their products.

Although General Foods does not have any allergy lists, the company does maintain a toll-free number for consumer questions. And to meet the needs of any consumer who believes he or she may have had an allergic reaction to one of their products, General Foods has a bonded employee who can access detailed information about proprietary flavorings in the event of an emergency.

ALLERGENS IN
BRAND-NAME FOODS

Food Item	CORN	EGGS	MILK	NUTS	PEANUT	SOY	WHEAT

A

Food Item	CORN	EGGS	MILK	NUTS	PEANUT	SOY	WHEAT
A-1 Steak Sauce	C		M				W
ALBA '77, Fit'N Frosty:							
Vanilla	C		M		P	S	
ALBACORE (See **TUNA**)							
ALMOND BUTTER:							
(Erewhon)				N			
(Walnut Acres)				N	P		
ALMOND MEAL:							
(Ener-G Foods) NutQuik				N			
ALMONDS, CAROB-COATED:							
(Walnut Acres)			M	N		S	
APPLE, CANDY:							
Coating Mix (Concord)	C						
APPLE, CARAMEL:							
Caramel Apple Wrap (Concord)	C		M				
Coating Mix (Concord)	C		M			S	W
APPLE, DRIED:							
Apple Snack (Weight Watchers)							
APPLE-GRAPE JUICE:							
(Mott's)							
APPLE JUICE:							
(Mott's)							
From Concentrate							
Natural							
(Red Cheek)							
From Concentrate							
Natural							
(Speas Farm)							
APPLE-RASPBERRY JUICE:							
(Mott's)							
APPLES, FROZEN:							
(Stouffer's):							
Escalloped Apples	C		M		P		W
Yams & Apples	C						W

Food Item	CORN	EGGS	MILK	NUTS	PEANUT	SOY	WHEAT
APPLESAUCE:							
(Mott's):							
Cinnamon	C						
Natural	C						
Regular	C						
(Very Fine) 100% McIntosh	C						
APRICOT NUT CAKE:							
(Walnut Acres)		E	M	N			W
APRICOTS, canned:							
(Del Monte), heavy syrup	C						
ARBY'S:							
Meats:							
Roast beef							
Turkey	C						
Sauces:							
Arby's	C						W
Cheddar Cheese	C		M			S	W
ARMOUR							
Dinner Classics, frozen meals:							
Boneless Beef Short Ribs	C		M			S	W
Chicken Fricassee	C		M			S	W
Chicken Milan	C		M	N	P	S	W
Salisbury Steak	C	E	M		P	S	W
Seafood Newburg	C	E	M		P	S	W
Sirloin Roast	C		M			S	W
Meats:							
Armour Star:							
Cured Fat Back							
Cured Salt Pork							
Chopped Ham	C						
Chopped Pork	C						
Cooked Ham, Bone-in	C						
Corned Beef Brisket, round							
Ham	C						
Pork Shoulder Picnic	C						
Spiced Luncheon Meat	C						
Vienna Sausage	C						
Golden Star Ham	C						
Hot Dogs	C						

Food Item	CORN	EGGS	MILK	NUTS	PEANUT	SOY	WHEAT
ARROWHEAD MILLS:							
Bread Mixes:							
Biscuit Mix	C		M				W
Bran Muffin	C		M			S	W
Corn Bread	C		M			S	W
Multigrain			M			S	W
Whole Wheat			M				W
Cake Mixes:							
Carob			M				W
Choice	C	E	M		P	S	W
Multi-Cake	C		M				W
Cereals:							
Bear Mush							W
4 Grain + Flax							W
Nature O's							W
Puffed:							
Corn	C						
Rice							
Wheat							W
Rice & Shine							
7 Grain	C					S	W
Pancake Mixes:							
Buckwheat	C		M				W
Griddle Lite	C	E	M		P	S	
Multigrain	C		M				W
Triticale	C		M				W
Peanut Butter:							
Creamy					P		
Crunchy					P		
Tamari Soy Sauce						S	W
ARROWROOT STARCH:							
(Premier Japan):							
Kuzu (wild arrowroot starch)							
ARTICHOKE HEARTS, marinated:							
(Cara Mia)	C					S	W
(Goya)	C					S	W
(Progresso)	C					S	W
ASPARAGUS, canned:							
(Del Monte) tips							
(Green Giant) spears							

Food Item	CORN	EGGS	MILK	NUTS	PEANUT	SOY	WHEAT
(White Rose) spears							
AUNT JEMIMA (See **SYRUP; PANCAKE MIX**)							
AVOCADO DIP, frozen:							
(Calavo)	C						

Food Item	C O R N	E G G S	M I L K	N U T S	P E A N U T	S O Y	W H E A T

B

BABA-AU-RHUM:
  (Ferrara)　　　　　　　　C　E　　　　　　S　W
BABY FOOD:
  (Beech-Nut):
    Cereals, Dry, Stage I:
      Barley　　　　　　　　　　　　　　　　　W
      Oatmeal　　　　　　　　　　　　　　　　W
      Rice　　　　　　　　　C　　　　　　P　S
    Cereals, Dry, Stage II:
      Hi-Protein　　　　　　　　　　　　　　S　W
      Mixed　　　　　　　　C　　　　　　　　W
      Oatmeal with Banana　C　　　　　　　　W
      Rice with Banana　　　C　　　　　　S
    Cereals, Jarred, Stage II:
      Mixed with Applesauce & Bananas　C　　　　　　　W
      Oatmeal with Applesauce &
        Bananas　　　　　　　C　　　　　　　　W
      Rice with Applesauce & Bananas　C　　M
    Desserts, Stage II:
      Banana Custard Pudding　　C　E　M
      Banana Pineapple Dessert　　C
      Cottage Cheese with Pineapple　C　　M
      Dutch Apple Dessert　　　C　　M
      Guava Fruit Dessert　　　C
      Mango Fruit Dessert　　　C
      Mixed Fruit & Yogurt　　C　　M
      Papaya Fruit Dessert　　C
      Peaches & Yogurt　　　　C　　M
      Vanilla Custard Pudding　C　E　M
    Desserts, Stage III:
      Banana Custard Pudding　　C　E　M
      Cottage Cheese with Pineapple　C　　M
      Mixed Fruit & Yogurt　　C　　M
      Peaches & Yogurt　　　　C　　M

Food Item	CORN	EGGS	MILK	NUTS	PEANUT	SOY	WHEAT
Vanilla Custard Pudding	C	E	M				
Dinners, Stage II:							
Beef & Egg Noodle	C	E					W
Beef Supreme	C		M				
Chicken & Rice							
Chicken Noodle	C	E					W
Macaroni, Tomato, & Beef		E	M				W
Turkey Rice							
Turkey Supreme	C						
Vegetable Beef							
Vegetable Chicken			M				
Vegetable Ham							
Vegetable Lamb							
Dinners, Stage III:							
Beef & Egg Noodle	C	E					W
Beef Supreme	C						
Chicken Noodle	C	E					W
Macaroni, Tomato, & Beef	C	E	M				W
Spaghetti, Tomato, & Beef	C	E	M				W
Turkey Rice							
Turkey Supreme	C						
Vegetable Bacon	C						
Vegetable Beef							
Vegetable Chicken	C		M				
Vegetable Lamb	C						
Fruits, Stage I:							
Applesauce	C						
Bananas	C						
Peaches	C						
Pears	C						
Fruits, Stage II							
Applesauce & Apricots	C						
Applesauce & Bananas	C						
Applesauce & Cherries	C						
Apricots with Pears, Apples	C						
Bananas with Pears, Apples	C						
Fruit Dessert	C						
Pears & Applesauce	C						
Pears & Pineapple	C						
Plums with Rice	C						

Food Item	C O R N	E G G S	M I L K	N U T S	P E A N U T	S O Y	W H E A T
Prunes with Pears							
Fruits, Stage III:							
Applesauce	C						
Applesauce & Bananas	C						
Applesauce & Cherries	C						
Apricots, Pears, Apples	C						
Bananas, Pears, Apples	C						
Fruit Dessert	C						
Peaches	C						
Pears	C						
Pears & Pineapples	C						
Fruit Supreme Desserts, Stage II:							
Apples & Grapes	C						
Apples, Oranges, Bananas	C						
Apples, Peaches, Strawberries	C						
Apples, Pears, Bananas	C						
Apples & Strawberries	C						
Island Fruits	C						
Fruit Supreme Desserts, Stage III:							
Apples & Grapes	C						
Apples, Oranges, Bananas	C						
Apples, Peaches, Strawberries	C						
Apples, Pears, Bananas	C						
Apples & Strawberries	C						
Island Fruits	C						
Juices, Stage I:							
Apple	C						
Grape	C						
Pear	C						
Juices, Stage II:							
Juice Plus, grape	C						
Juices, Unstaged:							
Apple	C						
Apple Banana	C						
Apple Cherry	C						
Apple Cranberry	C						
Apple Grape	C						
Apple Pear	C						
Mixed Fruit	C						
Orange	C						

Food Item	CORN	EGGS	MILK	NUTS	PEANUT	SOY	WHEAT
Tropical Blend	C						
Meats, Stage I:							
Beef							
Chicken							
Lamb							
Turkey							
Veal							
Vegetables, Stage I:							
Carrots							
Green Beans							
Squash							
Sweet Peas							
Sweet Potatoes							
Vegetables, Stage II:							
Creamed Corn	C		M				
Garden Vegetables							
Mixed Vegetables	C						
Peas & Carrots							
Vegetables, Stage III:							
Carrots							
Green Beans							
Mixed Vegetables							
Sweet Potatoes							
Table Time meals:							
Beef Stew	C		M				W
Chicken with Stars Soup	C	E	M				W
Pasta Squares in Meat Sauce	C	E	M				W
Spaghetti Rings in Meat Sauce	C	E	M				W
Vegetable Soup	C	E					
Vegetable Stew with Chicken	C		M				W
(Gerber):							
Baked Goods:							
Arrowroot Cookies	C		M			S	W
Cookies, Animal-shaped			M			S	W
Pretzels							W
Toddler Biter Biscuits	C		M			S	W
Zwieback Toast	C		M			S	W
Cereals, dry:							
Barley						S	W
High Protein						S	W

Food Item	C O R N	E G G S	M I L K	N U T S	P E A N U T	S O Y	W H E A T
Mixed	C					S	W
Oatmeal						S	W
Rice						S	W
Cereals with Fruit:							
High Protein with Apple, Orange	C					S	W
Mixed with Banana	C					S	W
Oatmeal with Banana	C					S	W
Rice with Banana	C					S	
Juices, 4.2 oz.:							
Apple	C						
Apple-Apricot	C						
Apple-Banana	C						
Apple-Cherry	C						
Apple-Grape	C						
Apple-Peach	C						
Apple-Pineapple	C						
Apple-Plum	C						
Apple-Prune	C						
Mixed Fruit	C						
Orange	C						
Orange-Apple	C						
Juices, 8 oz.:							
Apple	C						
Apple-Cherry	C						
Apple-Grape	C						
Apple'n Berry	C						
Apple-Pear	C						
Fruits-a-Plenty	C						
Fruits of the Sun	C						
Mixed Fruit	C						
Junior Desserts:							
Banana-Apple	C						
Cherry Vanilla Pudding	C	E					
Dutch Apple	C		M				
Fruit							
Hawaiian Delight	C		M				
Peach Cobbler	C						W
Vanilla Custard	C	E	M				W
Junior Dinners:							
Beef Egg Noodle		E					W

Food Item	CORN	EGGS	MILK	NUTS	PEANUT	SOY	WHEAT
Chicken Noodle		E					W
Macaroni & Cheese		E	M				W
Macaroni & Tomato with Beef		E	M				W
Spaghetti with Tomato Sauce & Beef		E	M			S	W
Split Pea & Ham			M				W
Turkey Rice							W
Vegetable Bacon			M			S	
Vegetable Beef							W
Vegetable Chicken						S	W
Vegetable Ham							W
Vegetable Lamb							W
Vegetable Turkey							W
Junior Fruits:							
Apple-Blueberry	C						
Applesauce	C						
Applesauce Apricot	C						
Apricots with Tapioca	C						
Banana with Tapioca	C						
Banana with Tapioca, Pineapple	C						
Peaches	C						
Pears	C						
Pear Pineapple	C						
Plums with Tapioca							
Junior High-Meat Dinners:							
Beef with Vegetables							W
Chicken with Vegetables							W
Ham with Vegetables							W
Turkey with Vegetables			M				W
Veal with Vegetables							W
Junior Jarred Cereals:							
Mixed with Applesauce, Banana	C						W
Oatmeal with Applesauce, Banana	C						W
Rice with Mixed Fruit	C		M				
Junior Meats:							
Beef							
Chicken							
Ham							
Lamb							
Turkey							

Food Item	CORN	EGGS	MILK	NUTS	PEANUT	SOY	WHEAT
Veal							
Junior Vegetables:							
Carrots							
Creamed Corn	C		M				
Creamed Green Beans			M				W
Mixed Vegetables							W
Peas							
Squash							
Sweet Potatoes							
Meat & Poultry Sticks:							
Chicken			M				
Meat			M				
Turkey			M				
Strained Desserts:							
Banana-Apple	C						
Cherry Vanilla Pudding	C	E					
Chocolate Custard	C	E	M				W
Dutch Apple	C		M				
Fruit	C						
Hawaiian Delight	C		M				
Orange Pudding	C	E	M				
Peach Cobbler	C						W
Vanilla Custard	C	E	M				W
Strained Dinners:							
Beef Egg Noodle		E					W
Cereal with Egg Yolk & Bacon	C	E	M				W
Chicken Noodle		E	M				W
Macaroni & Cheese		E	M				W
Macaroni & Tomato with Beef		E	M			S	W
Turkey Rice							W
Vegetable & Bacon						S	W
Vegetable & Beef							W
Vegetable & Chicken						S	W
Vegetable & Ham							W
Vegetable & Lamb							W
Vegetable Liver							W
Vegetable & Turkey							W
Strained Fruits:							
Apple Blueberry	C						
Applesauce	C						

Food Item	CORN	EGGS	MILK	NUTS	PEANUT	SOY	WHEAT
Applesauce & Apricots	C						
Applesauce with Pineapple	C						
Apricots with Tapioca	C						
Banana with Tapioca	C						
Banana with Tapioca, Pineapple	C						
Peaches	C						
Pear & Pineapple	C						
Pears	C						
Plums with Tapioca							
Prunes with Tapioca							
Strained High-Meat Dinners:							
Beef with Vegetables							W
Chicken with Vegetables							W
Ham with Vegetables							W
Turkey with Vegetables			M				W
Veal with Vegetables							W
Strained Jarred Cereals:							
Mixed with Applesauce, Bananas	C						W
Oatmeal with Applesauce, Bananas	C						W
Rice with Applesauce, Bananas	C		M				
Strained Meats & Eggs:							
Beef							
Beef Liver							
Chicken							
Egg Yolks		E					
Ham							
Lamb							
Pork							
Turkey							
Veal							
Strained Vegetables:							
Beets							
Carrots							
Creamed Corn	C		M				
Creamed spinach			M				W
Garden vegetables							
Green beans							
Mixed vegetables							W
Peas							
Squash							

Food Item	CORN	EGGS	MILK	NUTS	PEANUT	SOY	WHEAT
Sweet potatoes							
Toddler Foods:							
Beef & Egg Noodles		E				S	W
Noodles & Chicken		E				S	W
Potatoes & Ham	C		M				
Spaghetti with Tomato Sauce & Beef	C		M				W
Vegetables & Beef	C					S	W
Vegetables & Chicken						S	W
Vegetables & Ham						S	W
Vegetables & Turkey						S	W
(Health Valley Foods):							
Cereal:							
Instant Brown Rice							W
Sprouted Cereal with Bananas							W
BACARDI:							
Mai Tai Punch, frozen	C						
BACON:							
(Armour):							
Pan-Size	C						
Regular	C						
Thick sliced	C						
(Hormel):							
Black Label							
Canadian-style			M			S	W
Old Smokehouse			M			S	W
(*Range Brand*)							
Red Label			M				
Salt Pork			M				
(Oscar Mayer):							
Bacon Bits							
Center Cut							
Regular							
Thick Slice							
(Hygrade's):							
West Virginia	C						
(Thorn Apple Valley):							
Hickory Smoked	C						
(Wilson)	C						

Food Item	C O R N	E G G S	M I L K	N U T S	P E A N U T	S O Y	W H E A T
BACON, IMITATION:							
(Concord) Bacon Bits	C					S	W
BACON BITS:							
(Hormel)			M			S	W
(Oscar Mayer)							
BAGELS:							
(Lender's):							
Bagelettes:							
Onion	C						W
Plain	C	E					W
Bagels:							
Egg	C	E	M		P	S	W
Garlic	C						W
Onion	C						W
Plain	C						W
Poppy Seed	C						W
Pumpernickel	C		M				W
Raisin 'n Honey						S	W
Raisin 'n Wheat	C						W
Rye	C		M				W
Sesame Seed	C						W
(Sara Lee):							
Cinnamon & Raisin	C						W
Egg	C	E					W
Onion	C						W
Plain	C						W
Poppy Seed	C						W
BAKING MIX (See also **BISCUIT MIX;** **PANCAKE MIX**):							
(Ener-G Foods):							
Gluten-Free, Wheat-Free Mixes:							
Brown Rice Baking Mix	C			N			
Corn Mix	C						
Potato Mix							
Rice Mix							
Rice Mix, low sodium							
White Rice Baking Mix							
Wheat-free, with Gluten:							
Barley Mix							W
Oat Mix							W

Food Item	CORN	EGGS	MILK	NUTS	PEANUT	SOY	WHEAT
Rice 'N Rye Bread Mix							W
(Fearn):							
Brown Rice						S	
Rice						S	
(Welplan):							
Gluten-free:							
Potato and Corn Starch	C		M			S	
Regular, low-protein	C				P	S	W
BAKING POWDER:							
(Davis)	C						
(Ener-G Foods)							
(Walnut Acres)	C		M				
BAKING SODA:							
Arm & Hammer							
BANANA COATING MIX:							
(Concord) Chocolate-flavored	C	E	M		P	S	
BANANA CREAM PIE:							
Mix (Concord)	C		M		P	S	W
BARBECUE SAUCE:							
Thick & Rich (Hunt's):							
New Orleans Style	C			N			W
Original Recipe	C						W
(Walnut Acres)	C						W
BEAN SALAD:							
Three Bean (Hanover), Deli-style	C					S	W
BEANS, AZUKI:							
(Premier Japan)							
BEANS, BAKED:							
(B&M) Brick Oven:							
Barbecue	C						W
Regular							
(Campbell's) Pork & Beans	C						W
(Health Valley Farms):							
Boston-style							
Vegetarian with Miso						S	W
(Hormel):							
Beans & Bacon	C					S	W
Beans & Ham	C					S	W
Beans & Wieners	C					S	W
(Van Camp's) Pork & Beans	C						W

Food Item	C O R N	E G G S	M I L K	N U T S	P E A N U T	S O Y	W H E A T
(Walnut Acres):							
Beans & Hot Dogs							
BEANS, GARBANZO, canned:							
Old El Paso							
(Progresso)							
BEANS, GREEN:							
Canned:							
(Libby's) Natural Pack							
Frozen:							
(Birds Eye) Italian Green Beans							
BEANS, KIDNEY, canned:							
(Progresso)							
BEANS, MEXICAN:							
Old El Paso:							
Mexe-Beans							
Pinto Beans							
Refried Beans							
BEANS, RED, canned:							
(Goya) Small Red Beans							
BEEF, CREAMED DRIED:							
(Hormel)	C		M			S	W
BEEF, FROZEN:							
(Quaker Maid):							
Beef Patties							
Breaded Beef & Veal Patties						S	
Italian Meatballs	C		M			S	W
Sandwich Slices						S	
Sandwich Steaks							
BEEF, PREPARED:							
(De Witt's Table Ready Meats):							
Rib Eye Roasts	C		M			S	W
Rib Eye Steaks	C		M			S	W
Strip Loin Steaks	C		M			S	W
Top Round Roasts	C		M			S	W
Top Round Steaks	C		M			S	W
BEEF ENTRÉES, canned:							
Dinty Moore:							
Beef Stew	C					S	
(Hormel):							
Beef Goulash	C		M			S	W

Food Item	CORN	EGGS	MILK	NUTS	PEANUT	SOY	WHEAT
Beef Tamales	C		M			S	
Old El Paso:							
Beef Enchiladas	C					S	W
Beef Taco Filling	C		M			S	W
(Walnut Acres):							
Beef Stew			M				W
Braised Beef Hash							
BEEF ENTRÉES, frozen:							
(Armour) *Dinner Classics:*							
Boneless Beef Short Ribs	C		M			S	W
Salisbury Steak	C	E	M		P	S	W
Sirloin Roast	C		M			S	W
(Myers):							
Beef Pie	C		M		P	S	W
Beef Stroganoff with Noodles	C	E	M			S	W
Creamed Chipped Beef	C		M		P	S	W
Macaroni & Beef	C					S	W
(Stouffer's):							
Creamed Chipped Beef	C		M				W
BILMAR (See **TURKEY**)							
BISCUIT MIX (See also **BAKING MIX**):							
(Arrowhead Mills)	C		M				W
(General Mills) *Bisquick*			M			S	W
BLINTZES:							
(Golden):							
Cheese	C	E	M		P	S	W
Potato	C	E			P	S	W
BOLOGNA (See also **LUNCHEON MEAT**):							
(Hormel):							
Coarse Ground	C		M			S	
Coarse Ground, Beef Bologna	C		M			S	W
Fine Ground	C		M			S	
(Hygrade's):							
Chicken *Grillmaster*	C						
BORSCHT:							
(Manischewitz):							
Low-calorie	C						
With Beets	C						

Food Item	CORN	EGGS	MILK	NUTS	PEANUT	SOY	WHEAT
BRAN:							
(Kretschmer) Toasted							W
(Quaker) Unprocessed							W
BRAUNSCHWEIGER							
(See **LIVERWURST**):							
BREAD (See also **Rolls**):							
(Arnold):							
Bran'nola, Hearty Wheat	C	E	M		P	S	W
Brick Oven White	C		M		P	S	W
Milk & Honey, Oatmeal	C	E	M		P	S	W
(Ener-G Foods):							
Brown Rice				N			
Hamburger Buns:							
Brown Rice				N			
White Rice							
Hotdog Buns, White Rice							
Rice Cinnamon Rolls	C					S	
Rice & Fiber	C					S	
Rice Starch	C		M			S	
White Rice							
Xanthan	C	E				S	
Yeast-Free Rice	C						
Grossinger's:							
Onion Rye	C		M		P	S	W
Pumpernickel	C		M		P	S	W
Rye, no seeds	C		M		P	S	W
Rye, seeds	C		M		P	S	W
Home Pride, Butter Top White	C		M		P	S	W
(Pepperidge Farm):							
Family Wheat	C	E	M		P	S	W
Honey Bran	C	E	M		P	S	W
Oatmeal	C	E	M		P	S	W
Raisin with Cinnamon	C	E	M		P	S	W
Sandwich, White	C	E	M		P	S	W
Wheat	C				P	S	W
White, thin-sliced	C	E	M		P	S	W
Whole Wheat, thin-sliced	C	E	M		P	S	W
(Sun Maid):							
Cinnamon Raisin Swirl	C	E	M		P	S	W

Food Item	CORN	EGGS	MILK	NUTS	PEANUT	SOY	WHEAT
(Thomas'):							
Date Nut Loaf	C	E		N		S	W
Protein, fresh	C				P	S	W
Protein, frozen	C				P	S	W
Sahara, mini-loaf pita	C				P	S	W
Sahara, whole wheat pita	C						W
(Walnut Acres):							
Cornell Formula	C	E	M			S	W
Molasses Bran	C						W
Oatmeal Hearth	C	E					W
Raisin	C		M				W
Raisin Bran	C						W
Rye	C		M				W
Soya Carob			M			S	W
12-Grain	C	E				S	W
Whole Wheat	C		M				W
BREAD, CANNED:							
(Welplan) Brown Bread	C					S	
BREAD CRUMBS:							
(Ener-G Foods)				N			
(4 C) Redi-Flavored	C		M		P	S	W
(Progresso) Italian-style	C		M		P	S	W
BREAD DOUGH, FROZEN:							
White:							
(Bridgford)			M			S	W
(Rhodes) White	C		M		P	S	W
BREAD MIX (See also MUFFINS):							
(Arrowhead Mills):							
Biscuit Mix	C		M				W
Corn Bread	C		M			S	W
Multigrain			M			S	W
Whole Wheat			M				W
(Dromedary) Corn	C					S	W
(Fearn):							
Corn Bread	C		M			S	W
(Home Hearth):							
French							W
Old Fashioned White			M			S	W
Rye			M			S	W
New World	C					S	W

Food Item	CORN	EGGS	MILK	NUTS	PEANUT	SOY	WHEAT
(Walnut Acres):							
Apricot Nut	C		M	N		S	W
Banana Nut	C		M	N		S	W
Date Nut	C		M	N		S	W
High Lysine Corn	C		M				W
Spicy Apple Nut	C		M	N		S	W
Wheat-free Raisin Cinnamon	C		M			S	W
(Welplan)							
Potato & Corn Starch	C		M			S	
Potato, Corn Starch & Soya Bran	C		M			S	
Whole Wheat:							
(Arrowhead Mills)			M				W
BREAKFAST BARS:							
(Carnation):							
Chocolate Chip	C		M		P	S	W
BREAKFAST STRIPS:							
(Oscar Mayer) *Lean 'N Tasty:*							
Beef						S	
Pork						S	
BROTH, CANNED (See also **SOUP**):							
Chicken:							
(Swanson)	C					S	W
(College Inn)	C					S	W
BROTH, INSTANT:							
(Herb-Ox):							
Beef, low sodium	C		M			S	W
Chicken, low sodium	C					S	W
(MBT) Chicken	C					S	W
BROWNIE MIX:							
(Betty Crocker) Fudge	C	E	M		P	S	W
(Duncan Hines)							
Milk Chocolate	C		M			S	W
Mint Chocolate	C					S	W
Peanut Butter	C				P	S	W
Regular	C					S	W
(Pillsbury) Deluxe Fudge	C						W
BROWNIES:							
(Charles) Fudge Nut	C	E	M	N	P	S	W
BRUNSWICK STEW:							
Dinty Moore	C		M			S	W

Food Item	CORN	EGGS	MILK	NUTS	PEANUT	SOY	WHEAT
BUGLES (General Mills):							
Nacho Cheese	C		M		P	S	W
Regular	C				P	S	
BURGER KING:							
Beverages:							
Chocolate Shake	C		M		P	S	W
Diet Pepsi	C		M				W
Orange Juice							
Pepsi Cola	C		M				W
7-UP	C						
Strawberry Shake	C		M		P	S	W
Vanilla Shake	C		M		P	S	W
Breakfast items/Desserts							
Apple Pie	C	E	M		P	S	W
Egg Mix	C	E	M		P	S	
French Toast Sticks	C	E	M		P	S	W
Great Danish	C	E	M	N	P	S	W
Buns:							
Burger	C		M		P	S	W
Croissant	C	E	M		P	S	W
Specialty Sandwich	C		M		P	S	W
Whopper	C		M		P	S	W
Condiments:							
Barbecue Sauce	C					S	W
Horseradish Sauce	C	E				S	W
Ketchup	C						W
Mayonnaise	C	E				S	W
Mustard	C						W
Sweet & Sour Sauce	C					S	W
Tartar Sauce	C	E				S	W
Meat, Fish, Poultry:							
Bacon	C						
Burger Patty							
Chicken Specialty	C		M		P	S	W
Chicken Tenders	C		M		P	S	W
Ham	C						
Sausage	C					S	W
Whaler Fish Fillet	C		M		P	S	W
Whopper Patty							

Food Item	C O R N	E G G S	M I L K	N U T S	P E A N U T	S O Y	W H E A T
Salad Dressings:							
Blue Cheese	C	E	M			S	W
House	C	E	M			S	W
Italian, reduced calorie	C					S	W
Thousand Island	C	E				S	W
Sandwich Toppings:							
Cheese, American	C	E	M		P	S	
Lettuce							
Onion							
Pickles	C						W
Tomato							
Side Orders, fried:							
French Fries	C				P	S	
Hash Browns	C				P	S	
Onion Rings	C		M		P	S	W
BURRITO, frozen:							
(Old El Paso) Beef & Bean, Hot	C		M		P	S	W
BUTTERSCOTCH MORSELS:							
(Nestlé)	C	E	M		P	S	

Food Item	CORN	EGGS	MILK	NUTS	PEANUT	SOY	WHEAT

C

CALCIUM CARBONATE:
(Ener-G Foods)
CALCIUM CHLORIDE:
(Ener-G Foods)
CAKE, frozen:
Carrot Cake:

	C	E	M	N	P	S	W
(Oregon Farms)	C	E	M	N	P	S	W

Cheesecake, Cream Cheese:

| (Sara Lee) | C | E | M | | | S | W |
| *R.S.V.P.* | C | E | M | | P | S | W |

Chocolate Hazelnut:

| (Oregon Farms) | C | E | M | N | P | S | W |

Coffee Cake:

| (Sara Lee) Streusel | C | E | M | | P | S | W |

Crumb Cake:
(Oregon Farms):

| Blueberry | C | E | M | | P | S | W |
| French Crumb | C | E | M | | P | S | W |

Cupcakes:

| (Oregon Farms) Yellow | C | E | M | | P | S | W |

Danish Pastry:

| Cheese (Sara Lee) | C | E | M | | P | S | W |

Layer Cake:
(Pepperidge Farm):

| Chocolate Fudge | C | E | M | | P | S | W |
| Golden | C | E | M | | P | S | W |

Pound Cake:

| (Sara Lee) | C | E | M | | P | S | W |

CAKE, ready-to-eat:
Apple:
(Entenmann's):

Apple Puffs	C	E	M		P	S	W
Fruit Topped Buns, Apple	C	E	M		P	S	W
Apricot Nut (Walnut Acres)		E	M	N			W

Food Item	CORN	EGGS	MILK	NUTS	PEANUT	SOY	WHEAT
Banana:							
(Entenmann's):							
Banana Crunch Cake	C	E	M		P	S	W
Butter Sunshine (Entenmann's)	C	E	M		P	S	W
Cheese Topped Buns (Entenmann's)	C	E	M		P	S	W
Chocolate:							
(Freihofer's):							
Chocolate Party Cake	C	E	M		P	S	W
Chocolate Round Cake	C	E	M		P	S	W
Chocolate Chip:							
(Entenmann's):							
Chocolate Chip Crumb Loaf	C	E	M		P	S	W
Filled Chocolate Chip Crumb	C	E	M		P	S	W
Citrus:							
(Freihofer's) Citrus Ring	C	E	M		P	S	W
Coffee Cake:							
(Ener-G Foods):							
Apple-filled	C		M			S	
Raspberry-filled	C		M			S	
(Entenmann's):							
Apple Raisin Coffee Cake	C	E	M	N	P	S	W
Bavarian Creme Coffee Cake	C	E	M		P	S	W
Cheese Coffee Cake	C	E	M		P	S	W
Crumb Coffee Cake	C	E	M	N	P	S	W
Danish:							
(Entenmann's):							
Apricot Danish Twist	C	E	M	N	P	S	W
Cherry Cheese Danish	C	E	M		P	S	W
Cinnamon Danish Twist	C	E	M	N	P	S	W
Danish Coconut Tea Ring	C	E	M	N	P	S	W
Danish Ring	C	E	M		P	S	W
Sunshine Orange Danish Ring	C	E	M	N	P	S	W
Fruitcake:							
(Ener-G Foods)	C	E		N		S	
(Walnut Acres)	C	E	M	N			W
Lemon Filled French Crumb							
(Entenmann's)	C	E	M	N	P	S	W
Marshmallow Iced Devil's Food							
(Entenmann's)	C	E	M		P	S	W

Food Item	CORN	EGGS	MILK	NUTS	PEANUT	SOY	WHEAT
Old Fashioned Apple Strudel (Entenmann's)	C	E	M		P	S	W
Raisin Loaf (Entenmann's)	C	E	M		P	S	W
Swiss Cake Rolls *Little Debbie*	C	E	M		P	S	W
CAKE, refrigerated:							
Cheesecake *Baby Watson:*							
Blueberry	C	E	M				W
Chocolate		E	M				W
Pineapple	C	E	M				W
Plain		E	M				W
Strawberry	C	E	M				W
CAKE MATE, prepared frosting:							
Glossy Red	C		M				W
Glossy White, decorating gel	C						
CAKE MIXES:							
Angel:							
(Duncan Hines)	C	E			P	S	W
(Arrowhead Mills):							
Choice Cake Mix	C		M			S	W
Multi-Cake Mix	C		M				W
Banana:							
(Fearn)	C	E	M		P	S	W
Carob:							
(Arrowhead Mills)			M				W
(Fearn)	C	E	M		P	S	W
Carrot:							
(Betty Crocker) *Cake Lover's*	C		M	N	P	S	W
(Duncan Hines) Deluxe	C				P	S	W
(Fearn)	C	E	M		P	S	W
Chocolate Chip:							
(Betty Crocker)	C	E			P	S	W
(Duncan Hines)	C	E			P	S	W
Devil's Food:							
(Betty Crocker) *Supermoist*	C		M		P	S	W
(Duncan Hines) Deluxe	C				P	S	W
Fudge:							
(Duncan Hines) Butter Recipe	C				P	S	W
Gingerbread:							
(Betty Crocker) *Classics*	C				P	S	W
(Dromedary)		E				S	W

Food Item	CORN	EGGS	MILK	NUTS	PEANUT	SOY	WHEAT
Golden:							
(Duncan Hines) Butter Recipe	C				P	S	W
Pound Cake:							
(Dromedary)						S	W
Spice:							
(Fearn)	C	E	M		P	S	W
White:							
(Duncan Hines) Deluxe	C				P	S	W
Yellow:							
(Duncan Hines) Deluxe	C				P	S	W
CAKE MIXES, artificially sweetened:							
(Sweet 'n Low):							
Banana	C	E	M		P	S	W
Chocolate	C	E	M		P	S	W
Gingerbread	C	E	M		P	S	W
Lemon	C	E	M		P	S	W
Mint Chocolate	C	E	M		P	S	W
White	C	E	M		P	S	W
Yellow	C	E	M		P	S	
CAMPBELL'S (See also **SOUPS**):							
Chunky Soups:							
Clam Chowder, Manhattan-style	C					S	W
Sirloin Burger	C		M		P	S	W
Vegetable Beef, low sodium	C		M		P	S	
Condensed Soups:							
Chicken Barley	C		M			S	W
Chicken Broth & Rice	C					S	W
Cream of Asparagus	C		M			S	W
Cream of Celery	C		M			S	W
Cream of Chicken	C		M		P	S	W
Cream of Shrimp	C		M			S	W
Creamy Chicken Mushroom	C		M		P	S	W
Creamy Natural:							
Asparagus	C		M				W
Broccoli	C	E	M				W
Potato	C		M				W
Spinach	C		M				W
French Onion	C		M			S	W
Golden Mushroom	C					S	W
Oyster Stew	C		M			S	W

Food Item	CORN	EGGS	MILK	NUTS	PEANUT	SOY	WHEAT
Pepper Pot	C		M		P	S	W W
Zesty Tomato	C						W
CANDY:							
Almond, chocolate covered:							
(Hershey's) *Golden Almond*			M	N		S	
Almond Joy (Peter Paul)	C	E	M	N	P	S	
Andes:							
Creme de Menthe	C	E	M		P	S	
Mint Parfait	C	E	M		P	S	
Bingo Caramels & Taffy Squares							
(Switzer Clark)	C		M			S	
Black Cow (Switzer Clark)	C		M		P	S	
Black Jack (Switzer Clark)	C		M			S	W
Bonkers! Fruit Candy:							
Grape	C						
Orange	C						
Strawberry	C						
Watermelon	C						
Breath Savers, sugar free:							
Cinnamon	C						
Peppermint	C						
Spearmint	C						
Butter Mints (Charles)	C	E	M		P	S	
Butter Nut (Hollywood)	C		M		P	S	
Butterfinger	C		M		P	S	
Candy Corn:							
(*Heide*) with honey	C	E				S	
Caramello (Cadbury's)	C	E	M		P	S	
Cherries, chocolate-covered:							
(Cella's)	C					S	
Cortina (Welch's):							
Milk chocolate	C		M			S	
Dark chocolate	C					S	
Chew-ets (Goldenberg's)	C		M		P	S	
Chocolate:							
Chocolate, dark:							
Special Dark (Hershey's)						S	
Chocolate, milk:							
(Hershey's)			M			S	

Food Item	C O R N	E G G S	M I L K	N U T S	P E A N U T	S O Y	W H E A T
(Nabisco) Chocolate Stars			M			S	
(Nestlé)	C	E	M		P	S	
(Switzer Clark)			M			S	
Chocolate, milk, with Almonds							
(Hershey's)			M	N		S	
(Nestlé)	C	E	M	N	P	S	
Chocolate, white:							
Alpine White with Almonds							
(Nestlé)			M	N			
Chocolate Babies (Heide)	C	E				S	
Chocolate-covered Almonds:							
(Banner)	C	E		N	P	S	
Chocolate Egg (Hershey's)			M			S	
Chocolate Mint Perfects (Charles)	C	E	M		P	S	
Chocolaty Pay Day (Hollywood)	C	E	M		P	S	
Chuckles:							
Fruit Jellies	C						
Jelly Candy Bar	C						
Jelly Rings	C						
Ju Jubes	C						
Orange Slices	C						
Spearmint Leaves	C						
Spice Sticks & Drops	C						
Circus Peanuts (Brach's)	C					S	W
Clark bar	C	E	M		P	S	W
Conversation Hearts (Brach's)	C				P	S	W
Cough drops:							
(Beech-Nut)	C						
(Luden's):							
Honey Lemon	C						
Wild Cherry	C						
Pine Brothers:							
Assorted	C						
Honey	C						
Wild Cherry	C						
Creme Eggs (Cadbury's)	C	E	M			S	
Crispy (Switzer Clark)			M			S	
Crunch Bars (Nestlé)	C	E	M		P	S	W
Dessert Mints, assorted (Brach's)	C				P	S	W W
Dots (Mason)	C						W

Food Item	C O R N	E G G S	M I L K	N U T S	P E A N U T	S O Y	W H E A T
Drops (Heide)	C						
(Erewhon):							
Barley							W
Cinnamon							W
Ginger							W
Peppermint							W
Plum							W
Ume							W
Fanfare (Mars)	C	E	M	N	P	S	
Fifth Avenue (Ludens)	C	E	M	N	P	S	
Fruit Choos (Switzer Clark)	C					S	
Fruit Drops (Charles)	C						
Goobers (Nestlé)	C	E	M		P	S	
Good & Fruity (Switzer Clark)	C				P	S	W
Good & Plenty (Switzer Clark)	C		M				W
Gummi Bears (Heide)	C						
Gummi Hearts of Gold (Stark)	C					S	W
Hot Tamales (Just Born)	C						W
Jawbreakers (Willy Wonka's):							
DinaSour Eggs	C				P	S	W
Everlasting Gobstopper	C				P	S	W
Rinky Dinks	C				P	S	W
Jelly Beans:							
(Heide) Jelly Eggs	C						
(Jelly Belly) Very Cherry	C						
(Maillard):							
Petite Pectin Jelly Eggs	C						W
Teenee Beanees	C						W
(Rodda) Jelly Eggs	C						W
Jolly Joes (Just Born)	C						W
(Jolly Rancher) kisses, assorted	C						
Jujyfruits (Heide)	C						
Junior Mints	C						
Kisses (Hershey's)			M			S	
Kit Kat (Hershey's)			M			S	W
Krackel (Hershey's)			M			S	W
Licorice:							
(Panda)							W
(Switzer Clark), black:							
Bars	C		M				W

Food Item	CORN	EGGS	MILK	NUTS	PEANUT	SOY	WHEAT
Bites	C		M			S	W
Chewstrings	C		M				W
Ropes	C		M				W
Stix	C		M			S	W
Whips	C		M			S	W
(Switzer Clark), red:							
Bars	C						W
Chewstrings	C						W
Stix	C					S	W
Whips	C					S	W
(Y & S):							
Bites	C					S	W
Cherry Bits	C					S	W
Nibs	C					S	W
Twizzlers	C				P	S	W
Licorice Drops (Charles)	C						
Life Savers, roll candy:							
Butter Creme Mint	C		M				
Butter Rum	C		M				
Butterscotch	C		M				
Cin-O-Mon	C						
Cryst-O-Mint	C						
Fancy Fruits	C						
Five Flavor	C						
Pep-O-Mint	C						
Root Beer	C						
Spear-O-Mint	C						
Stik-O-Pep	C						
Strawberry	C						
Tangerine	C						
Tropical Fruits	C						
Wild Cherry	C						
Wint-O-Green	C						
Life Savers, sours	C						
Lollipops:							
(Charms):							
Blow Pops	C				P	S	W
Sweet Pops	C						
(Life Savers):							
Assorted	C						

Food Item	CORN	EGGS	MILK	NUTS	PEANUT	SOY	WHEAT
Carnival	C						
Swirled	C						
L's Jells (Luden's)	C						
M&M's (Mars):							
Holidays, peanut	C	E	M		P	S	W
Holidays, plain	C	E	M		P	S	W
Peanut	C	E	M		P	S	W
Plain	C	E	M		P	S	W
(Maillard):							
Assorted Jordan almonds				N			W
Bulk Chocolates:							
Chocolate Orange Peels	C	E			P	S	
Chocolate Rum Raisins	C	E			P	S	
Chocolate Strawberry Cordials	C	E			P	S	
Candy Coated Raisins						S	
Chocolate Almondolas			M	N		S	
Chocolate Apricot Brandy Cordials	C	E	M		P	S	
Chocolate Cherry Cordials	C	E	M		P	S	
Chocolate Coffee Beans	C	E	M		P	S	
Chocolate Covered Almonds	C	E	M	N	P	S	
Chocolate Covered Peanuts	C	E	M		P	S	
Chocolate Covered Raisins	C	E	M		P	S	
Chocolate Fruit & Nuts	C	E	M	N	P	S	
Chocolate Hazelnut Truffles			M	N		S	
Chocolate Mandarin Orange Cordials	C	E	M		P	S	
Chocolate Mint Almonds	C	E	M	N	P	S	
Chocolate Rum Cordials	C	E	M		P	S	
Chocolate Sesame Crunch	C	E	M		P	S	
Cocoa Almonds	C	E		N	P	S	
Eagle Sweet Chocolate	C	E			P	S	
Frosted Almonds	C	E	M	N	P	S	
Fruit Slices:							
Bulk	C	E			P	S	
12-oz. pkg.	C	E					
Lentils	C	E			P	S	W
Licorice Lentils	C	E	M		P	S	
Marzipan	C			N			
Mint Lentils	C	E			P	S	W
Mocha Lentils	C	E	M		P	S	

Food Item	CORN	EGGS	MILK	NUTS	PEANUT	SOY	WHEAT
Pastel Fruit & Nut				N	P	S	
Sea Shells							
Maple Sugar (Walnut Acres)							
Mars bar	C	E	M	N	P	S	
Marshmallow, novelties (Rodda):							
Bunnies	C					S	
Cats	C					S	
Peeps	C					S	
Pumpkins	C					S	
Snowmen	C					S	
Trees	C					S	
Marshmallow, toasted coconut:							
(Rodda)	C						
Mello Mint Peppermint Pattie	C	E			P	S	
Mentos (Van Melle), mixed fruit	C						
Mighty Bite (Switzer Clark):							
Apple	C					S	
Banana	C					S	
Cherry	C					S	
Grape	C					S	
Watermelon	C					S	
Mike & Ike (Just Born)	C						W
Milk Duds	C	E	M		P	S	W
Milk Shake (Hollywood)	C	E	M		P	S	W
Milky Way (Mars)	C	E	M		P	S	W
Mini Eggs (Cadbury's)	C	E	M		P	S	
Mints:							
(Richardson):							
After Dinner, jelly centers	C						
(Switzer Clark):							
Anise							
Assorted Jelly	C						
Butter			M				W
Pastel							
White							
Mr. Goodbar (Hershey's)			M		P	S	
Munch (Mars)	C	E	M		P	S	
Necco Wafers	C						
(Nestlé):							
Alpine White with Almonds			M	N			

Food Item	C O R N	E G G S	M I L K	N U T S	P E A N U T	S O Y	W H E A T
Crunch Bars	C	E	M		P	S	W
Milk Chocolate	C	E	M		P	S	
Milk Chocolate with Almonds	C	E	M	N	P	S	
Now & Later (Switzer Clark)							
Apple	C					S	
Banana	C					S	
Bubble Gum	C					S	
Cherry	C					S	
Chocolate	C		M			S	
Grape	C					S	
Mystery Mix	C					S	
Orange	C					S	
Pineapple	C					S	
Rainbow	C					S	
Raspberry	C					S	
Strawberry	C					S	
Tropical Punch	C					S	
Watermelon	C					S	
Nutcracker (Switzer Clark)			M		P	S	
Oh Henry! (Nestlé)	C	E	M		P	S	
One Hundred Grand (Nestlé)	C	E	M		P	S	W
Pay Day (Hollywood)	C	E	M		P	S	
Peanut Blossom Kiss (Switzer Clark)	C	E			P	S	W
Peanut Butter Frost (Ludens)	C	E	M		P	S	
Peanut Butter Logs (Switzer Clark)	C	E			P	S	
Peanut Chews (Goldenberg's)	C				P	S	
(Pearson's):							
Caramel Nip	C		M			S	
Chocolate Parfait	C		M			S	
Coffee Nip	C		M			S	
Coffioca Parfait	C		M			S	
Licorice Nip	C		M			S	
Mint Parfait	C		M			S	
Peppermint Patties (see also **THIN MINTS**):							
Mello Mint	C	E			P	S	
(Nabisco)	C	E				S	
York	C	E	M		P	S	
Perky jellies (Brach's)	C						W
Raisinets	C	E	M		P	S	

Food Item	CORN	EGGS	MILK	NUTS	PEANUT	SOY	WHEAT
Reese's:							
Peanut Butter Cups	C		M		P	S	
Reese's Pieces	C		M		P	S	
Rolo (Hershey's)	C		M			S	
Root Beer Barrels (Charles)	C						
Royals:							
Almond Chocolate	C	E	M	N	P	S	W
Cherry Cordial Chocolates	C	E	M		P	S	W
Irish Cream Chocolates	C	E	M		P	S	W
Mint Chocolates	C	E	M		P	S	W
Runts (Willy Wonka's)	C				P	S	W
(Russell Stover):							
Adelaides	C	E		N	P	S	
Almond Delights	C	E	M	N	P	S	
Butterscotch Squares	C	E	M		P	S	
Cherry Cordials	C	E			P	S	
Cherry Squares	C		M				
Coconut Clusters	C	E	M		P	S	
English Caramel, box	C	E			P	S	
French Chocolate Mints	C	E			P	S	
Fruit Flavored Jellies	C						
Honeysuckle Straws	C	E			P	S	
Lemon Squares	C	E	M		P	S	
Mint Patties	C	E			P	S	
Mint Squares	C	E	M		P	S	
Peanut Delights	C	E	M		P	S	
Pecan Delights	C	E	M	N	P	S	
Rosebud Mints	C	E	M		P	S	
Skittles (Mars)	C					S	W
Skor (Hershey's)			M	N		S	
Slo Poke (Switzer Clark)	C		M		P	S	
Snickers (Mars)	C	E	M		P	S	
Spearmint Drops (Charles)	C						
Starburst (Mars):							
Original	C					S	W
Strawberry	C					S	W
Sunshine pack	C					S	W
Tart 'n Tinys (Willy Wonka's)	C				P	S	W
Thin Mints, chocolate-covered:							
After Eight	C					S	

Food Item	CORN	EGGS	MILK	NUTS	PEANUT	SOY	WHEAT
Cortina (Welch's)	C	E				S	
Haviland (Borden)	C	E	M			S	
Three Musketeers (Mars)	C	E	M		P	S	W
Tic Tac, orange	C				P	S	W
Toffee (Heath)							
Original	C	E	M	N	P	S	
Soft n' Crunchy	C	E	M	N	P	S	
Tootsie Roll	C		M		P	S	
Tootsie Roll Bubble Pop:							
Cherry	C				P	S	
Grape	C				P	S	
Tootsie Roll Pop, Cherry	C		M		P	S	
Turtles (De Met's)	C		M	N		S	
Twix Cookie Bars (Mars):							
Caramel	C	E	M		P	S	W
Peanut Butter	C	E	M		P	S	W
Whatchamacallit (Hershey's)			M		P	S	W
Zag-Nut (Switzer Clark)	C	E			P	S	
Zero (Hollywood)	C	E	M	N	P	S	W
CANDY-MAKING INGREDIENTS:							
(Wilton):							
Candy color:							
Blue	C	E			P	S	
Green	C	E			P	S	
Orange	C	E			P	S	
Pink	C	E			P	S	
Red	C	E			P	S	
Violet	C	E			P	S	
Yellow	C	E			P	S	
Candy Melts	C	E	M		P	S	
Candy Wafer & Fondant Mix							
Center Mix:							
Cherry	C	E					
Chocolate Creme	C	E					
Creme	C	E					
Lemon	C	E					
Maple	C	E					
Marshmallow	C						
Orange	C	E					
Raspberry	C	E					

Food Item	CORN	EGGS	MILK	NUTS	PEANUT	SOY	WHEAT
Rum	C	E					
Strawberry	C	E					
Color Flow Mix		E					
CAROB:							
(Walnut Acres):							
Chips	C	E	M		P	S	
Powder							
Wafers	C	E	M		P	S	
CAROB-COATED SNACKS:							
(Walnut Acres):							
Carob Almonds			M	N		S	
Carob Peanuts			M		P	S	
Carob Raisins			M			S	
CASHEW BUTTER:							
(Erewhon)				N			
CASHEWS (See **NUTS**)							
CASSEROLES, FROZEN:							
(Health Valley Foods)							
Lean Living Dinners:							
Spinach-Mushroom Casserole		E	M				W
CATSUP (See **KETCHUP**)							
CEREAL, ready-to-eat:							
(Arrowhead Mills):							
Bear Mush							W
Bran Flakes	C						W
Corn Grits	C						
Cracked Wheat							W
Four Grain + Flax							W
Granola:							
Apple Amaranth	C			N		S	W
Arrowhead Crunch	C					S	W
Grainstay	C						W
Maple Nut	C			N			W
Nature O's							W
Seven Grain	C					S	W
Puffed:							
Corn	C						
Rice							
Wheat							W
Rice & Shine							

Food Item	CORN	EGGS	MILK	NUTS	PEANUT	SOY	WHEAT
7 Grain	C					S	W
(Ener-G Foods):							
Corn Bran	C						
Corn Germ Cereal	C						
Oat Bran							W
100% Rye Cereal							W
(Erewhon):							
Crispy Brown Rice:							
Low Sodium							W
Regular							W
Fruit 'n Wheat				N			W
Granola:							
Date Nut	C			N			W
Honey Almond	C			N			W
Maple	C			N			W
Number Nine, with Bran, no salt	C			N			W
Spiced Apple	C			N			W
Sunflower Crunch	C						W
Raisin Bran							W
Wheat Flakes							W
(General Mills):							
Cheerios	C						W
Golden Grahams	C		M				W
Honey Nut Cheerios	C			N			W
Kix	C						W
Trix	C						W
(Health Valley Foods):							
Amaranth:							
Regular	C						W
With Bananas	C			N			W
With Raisins	C						W
Bran:							
Regular							W
With Apples, Cinnamon							W
With Bananas							W
With Hawaiian Fruit							W
With Raisins							W
Granola (*Real*):							
Almond Crunch				N		S	W
Apple Cinnamon				N		S	W

Food Item	CORN	EGGS	MILK	NUTS	PEANUT	SOY	WHEAT
Hawaiian Fruit				N		S	W
Maple Nut				N		S	W
Raisin Nut				N		S	W
Healthy Crunch:							
Almond Date				N		S	W
Apple Cinnamon						S	W
Hawaiian Fruit				N		S	W
Hearts O' Bran:							
Apples & Cinnamon							W
Raisins & Spice							W
Lites:							
Brown Rice							
Golden Corn	C						
Golden Wheat							W
Miller's Bran Flakes							W
Orangeola:							
Regular						S	W
With Almonds, Dates				N		S	W
With Bananas, Coconut & Hawaiian Fruit						S	W
Sprouts 7:							
with Bananas, Hawaiian Fruit							W
With Raisins							W
Stone Wheat:							
Flakes							W
Raisin Bran Flakes							W
(Kellogg's):							
Applejacks	C						W
Cocoa Krispies	C		M			S	W
Corn Flakes	C						W
Corn Pops	C					S	
Crispix	C						W
Frosted Flakes	C						W
Frosted Krispies	C						W
Frosted Mini-Wheats	C						W
Froot Loops	C					S	W
Honey & Nut Corn Flakes	C				P	S	W
Honey Smacks	C		M			S	W
Marshmallow Krispies	C						W
Product 19	C						W

Food Item	CORN	EGGS	MILK	NUTS	PEANUT	SOY	WHEAT
Raisin Bran	C						W
Raisin Squares	C				P	S	W
Rice Krispies	C						W
Special K	C		M				W
(Kolln)							
Crispy Oats							W
Fruit 'n Oat Bran Crunch							W
Oat Bran Crunch							W
(Nabisco):							
100% Bran							W
Shredded Wheat							W
Shredded Wheat 'N Bran							W
Spoon Size Shredded Wheat							W
Team	C						W
Toasted Wheat and Raisins							W
(Organic Milling) *Back to Nature:*							
Almond Crisp	C			N			W
Apple Bran Crunch	C						W
Banana Crisp	C						W
Bulk Granola:							
Apple Blueberry			M			S	W
Apple Cinnamon			M			S	W
Apple Cinnamon Almond			M	N		S	W
Apple Cinnamon Cashew			M	N		S	W
Apple Raspberry			M			S	W
Banana Almond				N		S	W
Banana Cashew				N		S	W
Coconut Date						S	W
Hi-Pro	C		M	N		S	W
Honey						S	W
Honey Almond				N		S	W
Honey Almond Cashew				N		S	W
Honey Almond Flakes	C			N			W
Honey Banana Flakes	C						W
Honey Date						S	W
Honey Date Cashew				N		S	W
Honey Hawaiian						S	W
Honey Orange				N		S	W
Honey Raisin						S	W
Honey Raisin Flakes	C						W

Food Item	CORN	EGGS	MILK	NUTS	PEANUT	SOY	WHEAT
Maple Nut				N		S	W
Nuts Galore				N		S	W
Orange Almond				N		S	W
Raisin Date			M	N		S	W
Raisin Nut				N		S	W
Seven-Grain						S	W
Seven-Grain Sprouted Flakes	C						W
Wheat Free/Sugar Free	C			N		S	W
Granola:							
Apple Cinnamon Cashew			M	N		S	W
Honey						S	W
Honey Almond				N		S	W
Honey Date						S	W
Honey Hawaiian						S	W
Honey Raisin						S	W
Seven-Grain						S	W
Granola Flakes:							
Honey Almond	C			N			W
Honey Banana	C						W
Honey Raisin	C						W
Hi-Protein Branola:							
Cinnamon Apple	C		M			S	W
Honey	C				P	S	W
Honey Raisin	C				P	S	W
Honey Bran Crunch	C						W
Multi-Grain Hi-Pro	C		M	N		S	W
New World:							
Multi-Grain	C			N		S	W
Raisin Bran	C						W
Raisin Bran Crunch	C						W
(Post):							
Alphabits	C						W
(Quaker):							
Cap'n Crunch	C						W
Corn Bran	C						W
Honey Graham Oh's	C		M		P	S	W
Life	C					S	W
(Ralston):							
Bran Chex	C						W

Food Item	CORN	EGGS	MILK	NUTS	PEANUT	SOY	WHEAT
Cookie Crisp:							
Chip-flavor	C					S	W
Wafer-flavor	C						W
Corn Chex	C						W
Corn Flakes	C						W
Crispy Oatmeal & Raisin Chex	C					S	W
Crispy Rice	C						W
Donkey Kong	C						W
Donkey Kong Junior	C						W
40% Bran Flakes	C						W
Fruit Rings	C						W
Raisin Bran	C					S	W
Rice Chex	C						W
Sugar Frosted Flakes	C						W
Sugar Frosted Rice	C						W
Tasteeos	C						W
Wheat & Raisin Chex	C					S	W
Wheat Chex	C						W
Sun Country Granola							
With Almonds	C		M	N		S	W
With Raisins	C		M			S	W
With Raisins & Dates	C		M			S	W
(Walnut Acres):							
Granola:							
Apple Cinnamon					P		W
Date Coconut							W
Granny's				N	P		W
Malted Barley	C			N			W
Maple Almond				N	P		W
Super Apple			M	N			W
Super Banana			M	N			W
Unsweetened				N	P		W
CEREAL, hot, to be prepared:							
Cream of Rice (Nabisco)							
Cream of Wheat (Nabisco):							
Instant						S	W
Mix 'n Eat:							
Quick							W
Regular							W
Apple 'n Cinnamon						S	W

Food Item	CORN	EGGS	MILK	NUTS	PEANUT	SOY	WHEAT
Brown Sugar Cinnamon			M			S	W
Maple Brown Sugar			M			S	W
Original	C		M			S	W
Strawberry	C		M			S	W
(Erewhon):							
Barley Plus							W
Brown Rice Cream							
Oat Bran with Wheat Germ							W
Oatmeal:							
(Quaker):							
Instant	C		M				W
Old Fashioned							W
Quick							W
(Ralston):							
Quick							W
Regular							W
Red Bird (Organic Milling)							
Bulk Hot Cereal:							
Germade Farina							W
High Fiber Farina							W
High Protein Farina						S	W
Ralston Cereal:							
Quick							W
Regular							W
(Walnut Acres):							
Bran Flakes							W
Brown Rice Cream Cereal							
Danny's Porridge							W
Four Grain	C					S	W
Hearty	C		M			S	W
Indian Meal							W
12 Grain	C					S	W
CERVALAT:							
(Hormel) *Viking*			M				
CHEESE:							
American:							
(Borden) Cheese Food, slices	C		M				
(Land O' Lakes), 4-Quart			M				
Bleu *Alouette*			M				

Food Item	CORN	EGGS	MILK	NUTS	PEANUT	SOY	WHEAT
Brie *Alouette*:							
With Herbs			M				
With Mushrooms			M				
With Onions			M				
Cottage (Flav-O-Rich):							
4% Milk Fat	C		M		P	S	
1% Milk Fat	C		M		P	S	
Gourmandise Walnut (Bongrain)			M	N			
(*Laughing Cow*):							
Baby Bel:							
Mini			M				
Mini, part-skim			M				
Part-skim			M				
Regular			M				
Bonbel:							
Mini			M				
Regular			M				
Baby Cheddar			M				
Bonbino			M				
Edam			M				
Gouda			M				
CHEESE BALLS:							
(Kaukauna):							
Jalapeño			M	N			
Port Wine			M	N			
Sharp Cheddar			M	N			
CHEESE ENTRÉES, frozen:							
(Health Valley Foods)							
Lean Living Dinners:							
Cheese Enchiladas	C		M			S	
(Health Valley Foods)							
Meals For Two:							
Cheese Eggplant			M			S	W
Cheese Enchiladas	C		M			S	W
CHEESE LOGS:							
(Kaukauna):							
Country Swiss	C		M	N			
Sharp Cheddar			M	N			
Smokey/Sharp Double			M	N			

Food Item	C O R N	E G G S	M I L K	N U T S	P E A N U T	S O Y	W H E A T
CHEESE SPREAD:							
Alouette (Bongrain):							
French Onion	C		M			S	W
Garden Vegetable	C		M				
Garlic & Spices	C		M			S	W
Mild Blue	C		M			S	W
Zesty Pepper			M				
Laughing Cow (Bel Cheese):							
Blue	C		M				
Cheddar Wedges	C		M				
Hot Pepper	C		M				
Provolone	C		M				
Reduced Calorie	C		M				
Regular	C		M				
(Walnut Acres):							
Sandwich	C		M				W
Smoked	C		M				W
CHEESE STICKS, frozen:							
(Farm Rich) Mozzarella	C	E	M			S	W
CHEESECAKE (See **CAKE**)							
CHERRIES, MARASCHINO:							
(Raffetto)							
CHESTNUTS, preserved:							
(Raffetto):							
Marrons in Brandy	C			N			
Marrons in Vanilla	C			N			
Marron Pieces in Vanilla	C			N			
Prepared Chestnuts				N			
CHICK PEAS (See **BEANS, GARBANZO**)							
CHICKEN, CANNED:							
(Hormel) Chunk:							
Breast of Chicken			M				
White & Dark Chicken			M				
CHICKEN, DICED, frozen (Tyson)							
CHICKEN, FRIED, frozen:							
(Swanson):							
White Portions Dinner	C	E	M		P	S	W

Food Item	CORN	EGGS	MILK	NUTS	PEANUT	SOY	WHEAT
(Weaver):							
Nuggets	C		M		P	S	W
Rondelets, original	C	E	M		P	S	W
CHICKEN, OVEN-READY:							
(Perdue):							
Breast Cutlets	C	E			P	S	W
Breast Nuggets	C	E	M		P	S	W
Breast Tenders	C	E	M		P	S	W
CHICK'N QUICK, frozen (Tyson):							
Breast Fillets	C	E	M		P	S	W
Breast Patties	C	E	M		P	S	W
Chicken Patties	C	E	M		P	S	W
Chick'n Chunks	C		M		P	S	W
Chick'n Chunks (Southern fried)	C		M		P	S	W
Chick'n Dippers	C		M		P	S	W
Chick'n with Cheddar	C		M		P	S	W
Swiss'n Bacon	C		M		P	S	W
Thick'n Zesty (Italian recipe)	C		M		P	S	W
CHICKEN ENTRÉES, canned:							
(Walnut Acres):							
Chicken Stew			M				W
CHICKEN ENTRÉES, frozen:							
(Armour) *Dinner Classics*:							
Chicken Fricassee	C		M			S	W
Chicken Milan	C		M	N	P	S	W
Teriyaki Chicken	C		M			S	W
(Health Valley Foods)							
Lean Living Dinners:							
Chicken à La King		E	M				W
Chicken Crepes		E	M				W
(Health Valley Foods)							
Meals For Two:							
Cheddar Chicken			M			S	W
Le Menu, frozen dinners:							
Chicken Cordon Bleu	C	E	M	N	P	S	W
(Myers):							
Chicken à la King	C		M		P	S	W
Chicken au Gratin		E	M				W
Chicken Pie	C		M		P	S	W

Food Item	CORN	EGGS	MILK	NUTS	PEANUT	SOY	WHEAT
(Myers) Cook-in-pouch:							
Chicken à la King	C		M		P	S	W
Chicken & Noodles	C		M		P	S	W
Chicken Parmigiana	C		M		P	S	W
Creamed Chicken	C		M		P	S	W
(Stouffer's):							
Chicken Pie	C	E	M				W
Creamed Chicken	C		M				W
Escalloped Chicken & Noodles	C	E	M				W
Lean Cuisine:							
Chicken Cacciatore	C	E	M		P		W
Chicken & Vegetables	C	E	M				W
(Tyson):							
Chicken à l'Orange	C		M	N	P	S	W
Chicken Cacciatore	C		M		P	S	W
Chicken Fiesta	C		M		P	S	W
Chicken Français	C		M	N	P	S	W
Chicken Marsala	C		M		P	S	W
Chicken Oriental	C		M		P	S	W
Chicken Parmigiana	C	E	M		P	S	W
Chicken Piccata	C		M		P	S	W
Chicken Sweet & Sour	C		M	N	P	S	W
CHILI, canned:							
(Health Valley Foods):							
Con Carne						S	W
Vegetarian with Beans							
Mild						S	W
Mild, no salt						S	
Spicy						S	W
Spicy, no salt						S	
With Lentils						S	
(Hormel):							
Chili, hot, with beans	C					S	W
Chili mac	C		M			S	W
Chili, no beans	C					S	W
Chili with beans	C					S	
(Old El Paso):							
Chili with Beans	C		M			S	W
(Walnut Acres):							
Chili Con Carne	C						

Food Item	CORN	EGGS	MILK	NUTS	PEANUT	SOY	WHEAT
CHILI MIX:							
(Fantastic)	C					S	W
(Tempo)	C						W
CHOCO-BAKE, (Nestlé)						S	
CHOCOLATE, BAKING:							
(Hershey's):							
Unsweetened							
CHOCOLATE CHIPS:							
(Baker's) Semi-sweet						S	
(Hershey's):							
Semi-sweet chips:							
Miniature			M			S	
Regular			M			S	
(Nestlé):							
Milk Chocolate Morsels	C	E	M		P	S	
Tollhouse, semi-sweet	C	E	M		P	S	
CHOCOLATE FUDGE TOPPING:							
(Hershey's)	C		M		P	S	
CHOCOLATE MILK:							
(Hershey's)	C		M				W
CHOCOLATE SYRUP (See SYRUP, Chocolate)							
CHOW MEIN, canned:							
(Hormel):							
Pork Chow Mein	C					S	W
CHOWDER (See SOUP)							
CHUTNEY:							
(Major Grey's) Mango	C						W
(Raffetto):							
Chut-Nut Colonial Chutney	C			N			W
Major Grey's Mango Chutney	C						W
Peach Ginger Chutney	C						W
CLAM SAUCE:							
Red:							
(Ferrara)	C					S	W
White:							
(Ferrara)	C					S	W
CLAMS, canned:							
(Doxsee), chopped							

Food Item	CORN	EGGS	MILK	NUTS	PEANUT	SOY	WHEAT
COCKTAIL MIX, prepared:							
(Giroux):							
Bloody Mary	C					S	W
Blue Hawaii	C						
Daiquiri	C				P	S	
Mai-Tai	C						
Margarita	C						
Old Fashioned	C		M				W
Piña Colada	C				P	S	W
Sweet & Sour	C	E					
Tom Collins	C						
Whiskey Sour	C						
Mi-Lem	C				P	S	
(Texas Best) Bloody Mary	C					S	W
COCOA:							
(Hershey's) unsweetened							
COCOA MIX, regular:							
(Carnation):							
Hot Cocoa	C		M			S	
Milk Chocolate	C		M			S	
Mint Hot Cocoa	C		M			S	
Rich Chocolate	C		M			S	
70-Calorie			M				
(Hershey's):							
Instant	C					S	
(Nestlé):							
Hot Cocoa	C		M			S	
With Mini-Marshmallows	C		M			S	W
(Swiss Miss):							
Milk Chocolate	C		M		P	S	
With Mini Marshmallows	C		M		P	S	W
COCOA MIX, sugar free:							
(Nestlé)			M				
(Swiss Miss)			M				
COCONUT:							
(Walnut Acres)							
COCONUT CREAM, canned:							
(Giroux)	C					S	W
COFFEE, INSTANT, flavored:							
(General Foods):							

Food Item	CORN	EGGS	MILK	NUTS	PEANUT	SOY	WHEAT
Double Dutch Chocolate	C	E	M		P	S	
COLESLAW DRESSING, MIX:							
(Concord)	C		M		P	S	
COMBOS:							
Cheddar Cheese	C	E	M		P	S	W
Cheese Crackers	C		M		P	S	W
Nacho Cheese	C	E	M		P	S	W
Pizza Cheese	C	E	M		P	S	W
CONES, Ice Cream:							
Comet (Nabisco):							
Cake-type						S	W
Chocolate flavored						S	W
Sugar Cones						S	W
COOKIE MIX, Artificially Sweetened:							
Chocolate Chip (Sweet 'n Low)	C	E	M		P	S	W
COOKIE MIX, Regular:							
Chocolate Chip:							
(Duncan Hines):							
Double Chocolate	C	E			P	S	W
Regular	C	E			P	S	W
Oatmeal:							
(Duncan Hines) Raisin			M			S	W
Peanut Butter:							
(Duncan Hines)	C				P	S	W
Sugar:							
(Duncan Hines) Golden			M			S	W
COOKIES:							
Almond:							
(Walnut Acres)			M	N			W
Anginetti (Stella D'Oro)		E			P	S	W
Anisette (Stella D'Oro):							
Sponge	C	E			P	S	W
Toast	C	E			P	S	W
Big Chip (Archway)	C	E			P	S	W
Breakfast Treats (Stella D'Oro)	C	E				S	W
Brownie Chocolate Nut							
(Pepperidge Farm)	C	E	M	N	P	S	W
Brussels Mint (Pepperidge Farm)	C	E	M	N	P	S	W
Butter:							
Butter Flavored (Sunshine)	C	E	M		P	S	W

Food Item	CORN	EGGS	MILK	NUTS	PEANUT	SOY	WHEAT
Chessmen (Pepperidge Farm)	C	E	M				W
Shuttle Cookies (Sunshine)	C	E	M		P	S	W
Caramel Patties (Interbake)	C	E	M		P	S	W
Carob Chip:							
(Walnut Acres)	C	E	M	N	P	S	W
Chips Deluxe (Keebler)	C	E	M		P	S	W
Chocolate Chip:							
(Archway)	C	E	M			S	W
(Duncan Hines):							
Butterscotch	C	E	M		P	S	W
Mint	C	E	M		P	S	W
Peanut Butter	C	E	M		P	S	W
Regular	C	E	M		P	S	W
Walnut	C	E		N	P	S	W
(Entenmann's)	C	E				S	W
(Freihofer's)	C	E				S	W
(Sunshine):							
Chip-a-roos	C	E	M		P	S	W
Chocolate	C		M		P	S	W
Chocolate Chunk Pecan							
(Pepperidge Farm)	C	E	M	N		S	W
Chocolate Fudge (Sunshine):							
Sandwich	C	E	M		P	S	W
Wafers	C	E	M		P	S	W
Chocolate Nuggets (Sunshine)	C	E	M	N	P	S	W
Coconut:							
(Walnut Acres)			M				W
Coconut Macaroon:							
(Charles) Bars	C	E			P	S	W
Cup Custard (Sunshine)	C	E	M		P	S	W
Date:							
(Walnut Acres) Nut			M	N			W
Dixie Vanilla (Sunshine)	C		M		P	S	W
(Ener-G Foods):							
Aglutella Vanilla-filled	C				P	S	
Chocolate Crisps	C		M			S	
Chocolate Sandwich	C					S	
Date, no sugar added		E					
Dutch Cocoa	C					S	
Lemon Sandwich	C					S	

Food Item	CORN	EGGS	MILK	NUTS	PEANUT	SOY	WHEAT
Lemon Shortbread	C					S	
Macaroons	C	E					
Orange	C					S	
Rice Carob	C	E				S	
Rice Chocolate	C	E			P	S	
Rice Peanut Butter	C	E	M		P	S	
Rice Spice	C	E				S	
Rice Walnut	C	E		N		S	
Fancy Tin (Sunshine)	C	E	M		P	S	W
Fig Bars:							
(Sunshine)	C	E	M		P	S	W
Vanilla (FFV)	C	E	M		P	S	W
Fudge:							
(Duncan Hines):							
Almond Fudge	C	E		N	P	S	W
Peanut Butter Fudge	C	E	M		P	S	W
Fudge Cremes (Keebler)	C	E	M		P	S	W
Fudge Sticks (Keebler)	C	E	M		P	S	W
Ginger:							
Ginger Man (Pepperidge Farm)		E				S	W
Ginger Snaps (Sunshine)	C		M		P	S	W
(Walnut Acres)			M				W
Gluten-Free (Wel-Plan):							
Chocolate Chip	C		M		P	S	
Cream Filled Cookies, chocolate	C			N	P	S	
Custard Cream	C			N		S	
Golden Raisin	C					S	
Half-coated with Chocolate	C		M		P	S	
Lincoln	C					S	
Low Protein Cream-Filled Wafers:							
Chocolate	C			N		S	
Vanilla	C			N		S	
Shortcake	C					S	
Sweet	C					S	
Golden Fruit (Sunshine)	C	E	M		P	S	W
GrandMa's (Frito-Lay):							
Fudge Chocolate Chip	C	E			P	S	W
Hazelnut (Pepperidge Farm)	C	E	M	N		S	W
(Health Valley Foods):							
Date Pecan			M	N			W

Food Item	C O R N	E G G S	M I L K	N U T S	P E A N U T	S O Y	W H E A T
Honey Jumbos:							
Cinnamon	C	E	M		P	S	W
Oatmeal			M			S	W
Peanut Butter	C	E	M		P	S	W
Oatmeal			M				W
Peanut Butter			M		P		W
Raisin Bran			M				W
Snaps:							
Animal			M			S	W
Carob			M				W
Cinnamon			M			S	W
Coconut			M				W
Ginger			M				W
Honey			M			S	W
Lemon			M				W
Yogurt			M				W
Hydrox (Sunshine):							
Double Scoop:							
Chocolate	C	E	M		P	S	W
Mint	C	E	M		P	S	W
Strawberry	C	E	M		P	S	W
Expanded filling	C	E	M		P	S	W
Jelly Tarts (FFV)	C		M			S	W
Lady Stella Assortment							
(Stella D'Oro)	C	E		N	P	S	W
Le Petit-Beurre (Lu)			M				W
Lemon Coolers (Sunshine)	C	E			P	S	W
Little Schoolboy (Lu)	C	E	M		P	S	W
Mallopuffs (Sunshine)	C				P	S	W
Mint:							
Mint Milano (Pepperidge Farm)	C	E	M		P	S	W
Mint Sandwich (FFV)	C	E	M		P	S	W
Thin Mints, *Girl Scout*	C		M		P	S	W
Molasses:							
(Archway) Old Fashion	C					S	W
(Walnut Acres)			M				W
(Nabisco):							
Almond Windmill	C	E	M	N		S	W
Almost Home:							
Apple Fruit Sticks	C		M			S	W

Food Item	CORN	EGGS	MILK	NUTS	PEANUT	SOY	WHEAT
Blueberry Fruit Sticks	C		M			S	W
Cherry Fruit Sticks	C		M			S	W
Double Chocolate Brownies	C	E	M			S	W
Fudge Chocolate Chip	C	E	M			S	W
Fudge Chocolate Chip Raisin	C		M			S	W
Fudge 'N Chocolate Chip Sandwiches	C	E	M			S	W
Fudge 'n Peanut Butter Chip	C	E	M		P	S	W
Fudge 'n Vanilla Creme Sandwiches	C	E	M			S	W
Iced Dutch Apple Fruit Sticks	C		M			S	W
Iced Oatmeal Raisin	C	E				S	W
Oatmeal Creme Sandwiches	C	E	M			S	W
Oatmeal Raisin	C	E	M			S	W
Peanut Butter Fudge Brownies	C	E	M		P	S	W
Real Chocolate Chip	C	E	M			S	W
Apple Newtons	C	E	M			S	W
Bakers Bonus:							
Oatmeal	C	E	M			S	W
Barnum's Animals	C		M			S	W
Biscos:							
Sugar Wafers	C		M			S	W
Waffle Cremes	C		M			S	W
Blueberry Newtons	C	E	M			S	W
Brown Edge Wafers	C		M			S	W
Bugs Bunny Grahams						S	W
Butter Flavored	C	E	M			S	W
Cameo Creme Sandwich	C		M			S	W
Chewy Chips Ahoy:							
Chocolate Chip	C	E	M			S	W
Pure Chocolate Chip	C		M			S	W
Chocolate Chip Snaps	C		M			S	W
Chocolate Grahams	C					S	W
Cookie Break:							
Mixed Creme Sandwich	C		M			S	W
Vanilla Creme Sandwich	C		M			S	W
Danish Butter Cremes			M			S	W
Devil's Food Cakes	C		M			S	W
Famous:							
Chocolate Wafers	C	E	M			S	W

Food Item	CORN	EGGS	MILK	NUTS	PEANUT	SOY	WHEAT
Fig Newtons	C		M			S	W
Fudge Chocolate Chip	C	E				S	W
Cookie 'n Fudge Striped							
Shortbread	C	E	M			S	W
Gaiety Fudge Sandwiches	C		M			S	W
Giggles Sandwiches	C	E				S	W
I Screams sandwiches:							
Chocolate	C		M			S	W
Vanilla	C		M			S	W
Ideal Bars, Chocolate Peanut	C		M		P	S	W
Imported Danish Cookies	C	E	M			S	W
Lorna Doone shortbread	C	E	M			S	W
Marshmallow:							
Puffs	C		M			S	W
Sandwich	C	E	M			S	W
Mayfair Assortment	C	E	M			S	W
Mystic Mint	C		M			S	W
National Arrowroot	C	E	M			S	W
Nilla Wafers	C	E	M			S	W
Nutter Butter:							
Sandwiches	C	E	M		P	S	W
Old Fashioned Ginger Snaps	C					S	W
Oreo:							
Double Stuf	C		M			S	W
Regular	C		M			S	W
Swiss Assortment	C		M			S	W
Swiss Creme	C		M			S	W
Pantry Molasses						S	W
Pinwheels	C					S	W
Pure Chocolate Middles	C	E	M			S	W
Social Tea	C	E	M			S	W
Super Heroes	C	E	M			S	W
Zwieback Toast		E	M			S	W
Oatmeal:							
(Archway)	C	E	M			S	W
(Charles), cream-filled	C		M		P	S	W
(Duncan Hines):							
Cinnamon	C	E			P	S	W
Raisin	C	E			P	S	W

Food Item	CORN	EGGS	MILK	NUTS	PEANUT	SOY	WHEAT
(Pepperidge Farm):							
Raisin		E				S	W
(Sunshine):							
Country Style	C				P	S	W
Peanut Sandwich	C				P	S	W
(Walnut Acres):							
Old Fashioned		E	M	N			W
Regular		E	M	N			W
Orange Milano (Pepperidge Farm)	C	E	M		P	S	W
Orleans (Pepperidge Farm)	C	E	M		P	S	W
Peanut Butter:							
(Duncan Hines):							
Peanut Butter Nut	C	E	M		P	S	W
(FFV) Sandwich	C	E	M		P	S	W
(Pepperidge Farm):							
Peanut Butter Chip	C	E	M		P	S	W
(Sunshine) Wafers	C	E	M		P	S	W
(Walnut Acres)		E	M		P		W
Pecan:							
(Walnut Acres) Maple			M	N			W
Sandwich:							
Chips 'n middles (Sunshine):							
Creme	C	E	M		P	S	W
Fudge	C	E	M		P	S	W
Mint	C	E	M		P	S	W
Peanut Butter	C	E	M		P	S	W
Shortbread:							
(Pepperidge Farm)	C	E	M			S	W
Sprinkles (Sunshine)	C	E			P	S	W
Striped Shortbread (Interbake)	C	E			P	S	W
Sugar Wafers:							
(Sunshine)	C	E	M		P	S	W
Sweetmeal (Peek Frean)	C		M		P	S	W
T.C. Rounds (Interbake)	C	E	M		P	S	W
Tango (Interbake)	C	E			P	S	W
Toy (Sunshine)	C		M		P	S	W
Trolley Cakes (FFV)	C	E	M		P	S	W
Tru Blu (Sunshine):							
Chocolate	C	E			P	S	W
Duplex Sandwich	C	E	M		P	S	W

Food Item	CORN	EGGS	MILK	NUTS	PEANUT	SOY	WHEAT
Lemon	C	E			P	S	W
Vanilla	C	E			P	S	W
Vanilla:							
(Barbara's) French Vanilla	C		M				W
(Sunshine) Wafers	C	E	M		P	S	W
Vienna Fingers (Sunshine)	C	E	M		P	S	W
Walnut (Walnut Acres):							
Black		E	M	N			W
Orange			M	N			W
Whole Wheat Bars (Interbake):							
Apple	C	E	M		P	S	W
Fig	C	E	M		P	S	W
Peach-apricot	C	E	M		P	S	W
Yum Yums (Sunshine)	C	E	M		P	S	W
CORN, canned:							
Del Monte, no salt	C						
(Green Giant) *Niblets*	C						
S & W	C						
CORN GERM:							
Naturfresh (Fearn)	C						
CORN BREAD MIX							
(See also **MUFFIN MIX**):							
(Arrowhead Mills)	C		M			S	W
CORN MEAL MIX:							
White:							
(Aunt Jemima), self-rising	C						W
CORNED BEEF HASH, canned:							
(Broadcast)							
Mary Kitchen						S	
COUSCOUS:							
(Fantastic)							W
(Near East)							W
Quick Pilaf (Fantastic Foods)	C					S	W
CRAB, DEVILED (Mrs. Paul's):							
Miniature	C		M		P	S	W
Regular	C		M		P	S	W
CRABAPPLES:							
(Raffetto) Spiced	C						W
CRACKERS							
(See also **NABISCO and SNACKS**):							

Food Item	CORN	EGGS	MILK	NUTS	PEANUT	SOY	WHEAT
Animal Crackers:							
(Charles)	C	E			P	S	W
(FFV)	C					S	W
(Ralston Purina)	C	E			P	S	W
(Sunshine)	C		M		P	S	W
Armenian Thin Bread (Venus)	C					S	W
Bran Wafers:							
Salt Free (Venus)						S	W
Brown Rice Crackers:							
(Premier Japan):							
Seaweed						S	
Sesame						S	
Brown Rice Snaps (Edward & Sons):							
Buckwheat/No Salt							W
Buckwheat/Tamari						S	W
No Salt/Sesame							
Onion/Garlic							
Tamari/Seaweed						S	
Tamari/Sesame						S	
(Bremner) Wafers							W
Cafe Crackers (Sunshine)	C		M		P	S	W
Cheddar:							
American Heritage (Sunshine)	C		M		P	S	W
(Charles)	C		M			S	W
Cheddar Snacks (Ralston)	C	E	M		P	S	W
Thins (Interbake)	C		M			S	W
Cheese & Chive (Ralston)	C	E	M		P	S	W
Cheese Flavored:							
Cheese Snacks (Ralston)	C	E	M		P	S	W
Cheez-It (Sunshine)			M		P	S	W
Cheese Peanut Butter:							
(Frito-Lay)	C		M		P	S	W
Cinnamon (Ener-G Foods)	C					S	
Corn Crackers:							
Salt-free (Venus)	C					S	W
Cracked Wheat Wafers:							
Salt-free (Venus)						S	W
Cracklesnax	C						W
Crispbread (Wasa), Lite Rye							W

Food Item	CORN	EGGS	MILK	NUTS	PEANUT	SOY	WHEAT
English Water Biscuits							
(Pepperidge Farm)			M			S	W
Gluten-free (Wel-Plan)	C				P	S	
Goldfish (Pepperidge Farm):							
Cheddar Cheese	C		M			S	W
Original			M			S	W
Pizza			M			S	W
Pretzel						S	W
Graham:							
Cinnamon (Sunshine)	C				P	S	W
Honey (Sunshine)	C				P	S	W
(Interbake) Regal	C	E			P	S	W
Sugar Honey (Ralston)	C	E			P	S	W
Ham 'n Cheese (Interbake)	C					S	W
(Health Valley Foods):							
Amaranth	C	E			P	S	W
Cheese Wheels			M				W
Herb	C						W
Honey Graham	C	E	M		P	S	W
Sesame	C						W
7-Grain, 7-Vegetable	C						W
Stoned Wheat	C						W
Wheat & Sweet Rye	C						W
Yogurt & Green Onion	C		M				W
Hi Ho (Sunshine)	C		M		P	S	W
Japanese (Erewhon):							
Brown Rice							
Brown Rice, Shoyu						S	W
Koishi						S	W
Nori Makai						S	W
(Manischewitz):							
Garlic Tams	C					S	W
Onion Tams	C					S	W
Tam Tams	C					S	W
Tam Tams, no-salt	C					S	W
Wheat Tams	C					S	W
(Nabisco):							
Better Blue Cheese			M			S	W
Better Cheddars			M			S	W
Better Nacho Cheese			M			S	W

Food Item	CORN	EGGS	MILK	NUTS	PEANUT	SOY	WHEAT
Better Swiss Cheese			M			S	W
Cheese:							
Nips			M			S	W
Peanut Butter Sandwiches	C		M		P	S	W
Ritz			M			S	W
Sandwich			M			S	W
Tid-Bit			M			S	W
Wheat Thins			M			S	W
Country Crackers	C		M			S	W
Cracker Meal							W
Crown Pilot						S	W
Dandy Oyster Crackers						S	W
Escort	C		M			S	W
French Onion Thins						S	W
Gitana Soda Crackers	C		M			S	W
Graham Cracker Crumbs	C					S	W
Graham Crackers	C					S	W
Great Crisps:							
Cheese n' Chive			M			S	W
French Onion	C	E	M			S	W
Nacho	C	E	M			S	W
Real Bacon			M			S	W
Savory Garlic			M			S	W
Sesame Snack	C		M			S	W
Tomato & Celery			M			S	W
Honey Maid Grahams	C					S	W
Nutty *Wheat Thins*	C	E		N		S	W
Oysterettes						S	W
Royal Lunch		E	M			S	W
Sea Rounds						S	W
Sesame Snack Thins	C		M			S	W
Sultana Soda Crackers	C					S	W
Trio Snack Thins	C		M			S	W
Twigs:							
Herb & Spice			M			S	W
Sesame & Cheese			M			S	W
Uneeda Biscuits						S	W
Waverly	C		M			S	W
Wheat Thins:							
Low salt	C					S	W

Food Item	CORN	EGGS	MILK	NUTS	PEANUT	SOY	WHEAT
Regular	C					S	W
Wheatsworth Stone Ground						S	W
Ocean Crisp (FFV)	C					S	W
Oyster:							
(Ralston)	C	E			P	S	W
(Sunshine)			M		P	S	W
Parmesan (Sunshine)	C		M		P	S	W
Pizza (Charles)	C		M			S	W
Pumpernickel (Sunshine)	C		M		P	S	W
Rich & Crisp (Ralston)	C					S	W
Rye:							
Rye Snacks (Ralston)	C	E			P	S	W
(Sunshine)	C				P	S	W
Rye Wafers:							
Salt-free (Venus)	C		M			S	W
RyKrisp (Ralston):							
Natural							W
Seasoned							W
Sesame							W
Saltines:							
Krispy (Sunshine)	C		M		P	S	W
Krispy, unsalted (Sunshine)	C		M		P	S	W
Lu (Burry)	C	E			P	S	W
(Ralston):							
Regular	C					S	W
Unsalted	C					S	W
Sesame & Wheat (Ralston)	C	E			P	S	W
Sesame Crisp (Interbake):							
Unsalted	C		M			S	W
Snackers (Ralston)	C					S	W
Soup and Oyster (Interbake)	C					S	W
Stone Creek (Burry):							
Cracked Wheat	C	E			P	S	W
Stoned Wheat (Interbake):							
Appetizer Crackers	C		M			S	W
Wafers	C		M			S	W
Town House (Keebler) low salt	C					S	W
Wheat:							
Appetizer (Interbake)	C					S	W
(Carr's) Whole Wheat						S	W

Food Item	CORN	EGGS	MILK	NUTS	PEANUT	SOY	WHEAT
(Sunshine)	C				P	S	W
Wheat Snacks (Ralston)	C	E			P	S	W
Wheat Wafers:							
(Sunshine)	C				P	S	W
Salt-free (Venus)						S	W
CRANAPPLE Juice (Ocean Spray)	C						
CRANBERRY JUICE COCKTAIL:							
(White Rose)	C						
CRANBERRY SAUCE:							
(Ocean Spray):							
CranRaspberry	C						
Jellied	C						
Whole Berry	C						
CREAM, WHIPPED (See **WHIPPED TOPPING**)							
CREAM PUFFS, frozen (Rich's):							
Bavarian Cream	C	E			P	S	W
CREAMER, nondairy:							
Coffee-Rich (Rich's)	C		M		P	S	
CREAMSICLES (Popsicle)	C		M		P	S	
CREAMY HEAD, cocktail foam	C				P	S	
CROISSANTS:							
Frozen:							
(Sara Lee):							
Butter		E	M				W
Cheese	C	E	M		P	S	W
Wheat 'n Honey	C	E	M		P	S	W
Packaged:							
(Pepperidge Farm):							
Sandwich Quartet	C	E	M		P	S	W
CROUTONS:							
(Ener-G Foods):							
Italian	C		M			S	
Plain	C					S	
(Pepperidge Farm):							
Onion & Garlic	C	E	M		P	S	W
Seasoned with Herbs & Cheese	C	E	M		P	S	W
CUPCAKES:							
(Hostess), Filled	C	E	M		P	S	W

Food Item	C O R N	E G G S	M I L K	N U T S	P E A N U T	S O Y	W H E A T
CURRY POWDER:							
(Javin) India Style	C						
CUSTARD MIX (See also **PUDDING & PIE FILLING**):							
Artificially sweetened:							
(Sweet 'n Low):							
Chocolate			M			S	
Lemon	C		M			S	W
Vanilla	C		M			S	W
Regular:							
(Jell-O) *Americana* Golden Egg	C	E	M				

Food Item	CORN	EGGS	MILK	NUTS	PEANUT	SOY	WHEAT

D

DATES:
  (Dromedary):
    Chopped
    Pitted
DE BOLE'S **PASTA** (See **PASTA**)
DEVILED HAM:

(Hormel)	C					S	
(Underwood)							

DEVILED *SPAM*
DE WITT'S *TABLE READY* **MEATS:**

Barbecue Turkey Breast							
Oven Roasted Turkey Breast							
Rib Eye Roasts	C		M			S	W
Rib Eye Steaks	C		M			S	W
Smoked Turkey Breast	C						
Strip Loin Steaks	C		M			S	W
Top Round Roasts	C		M			S	W
Top Round Steaks	C		M			S	W

DIP, canned:
  (Old El Paso):

Jalapeño Bean Dip	C						W
Taco Dip	C						W

DIP, mix:
  (Charles):

Country Garden	C					S	W
French Onion	C					S	W

  (Concord):

Vegetable	C					S	W

  (Edward & Sons) Miso Plus Dip Mix
    Ingredients:

Chive						S	
Jalapeño						S	

  (Pier Eight):

Country Style Bacon	C					S	W
Guacamole	C		M				W

Food Item	C O R N	E G G S	M I L K	N U T S	P E A N U T	S O Y	W H E A T
Onion Dill	C				P	S	W
DIP, prepared:							
(Flav-O-Rich):							
Bacon & Horseradish	C		M			S	W
French Onion	C		M			S	W
Jalapeño	C		M			S	W
(King Dip):							
French Onion	C		M		P	S	W
DOLE FRUIT 'N CREAM BARS:							
All flavors	C		M				
DOLE FRUIT 'N JUICE BARS:							
All flavors	C						
DOLE FRUIT SORBET (See **FRUIT SORBET**)							
DOLE WHIP, frozen confection:							
Banana	C	E	M		P	S	W
Lime	C	E	M		P	S	
Orange	C	E	M		P	S	
Pineapple	C	E	M		P	S	
Strawberry	C	E	M		P	S	
DOUGHNUTS:							
(Dutch Mill) Donut Holes:							
Chocolate-Dipped	C	E	M		P	S	W
Glazed		E	M			S	W
Sugared	C	E	M		P	S	W
(Ener-G Foods):							
Apple Flavor	C		M			S	
Banana	C		M			S	
Banana, Chocolate-Iced	C		M			S	
Plain, Chocolate-Iced	C	E		N		S	
Plain Rice	C	E		N		S	
Pumpkin	C					S	
Pumpkin, Chocolate-Iced	C					S	
(Entenmann's):							
Country Style Donuts	C	E	M	N	P	S	W
Devil's Food Crumb	C	E	M		P	S	W
Filled Donuts (Bavarian Creme)	C	E	M		P	S	W
Rich Frosted Donuts	C	E	M		P	S	W
(Pepperidge Farm)	C	E	M		P	S	W

Food Item	CORN	EGGS	MILK	NUTS	PEANUT	SOY	WHEAT
(Tastykake) Assorted:							
Cinnamon Sugar	C	E	M		P	S	W
Plain	C	E	M		P	S	W W
Powdered Sugar	C	E	M		P	S	W
DRAKE'S:							
Ring Ding Jr.	C	E	M		P	S	W
Yankee Doodles	C	E	M		P	S	W
DRINK MIX, artificially sweetened							
(See also **TEA, ICED**):							
Crystal Light:							
Caribbean Cooler	C						
Citrus	C						
Citrus Blend	C						
Fruit Punch	C						
Fruit Tea, Berry Flavor	C						
Grape	C						
Iced Tea with Lemon	C						
Lemon-Lime	C						
Tropical Fruit	C						
Fla-vor-aid sugar-free:							
Cherry	C						W
Grape	C						W W
Lemonade	C						W W
Tropical Punch	C						W
Sweet 'n Low:							
Cherry	C						
Fruit Punch	C						
Grape	C						
Lemonade	C						
DRINK MIX, regular:							
Country Time:							
Lemonade	C						
Pink Lemonade	C						
Kool-Aid:							
Mountain Berry	C						
Tropical Punch	C						
DRINK MIX, unsweetened:							
Fla-vor-aid unsweetened:							
Cherry	C						W
Grape	C						W W

Food Item	CORN	EGGS	MILK	NUTS	PEANUT	SOY	WHEAT
Lemon-Lime	C						W
Orange	C						W
Raspberry	C						W
Strawberry	C						W
Tropical Punch	C						W
Hawaiian Punch	C				P	S	
Kool-Aid, unsweetened:							
Cherry	C						
Sunshine Punch	C						

Food Item	CORN	EGGS	MILK	NUTS	PEANUT	SOY	WHEAT

E

ECLAIRS, frozen:

  (Rich's) Chocolate Eclairs:

	CORN	EGGS	MILK	NUTS	PEANUT	SOY	WHEAT
Bavarian Cream	C	E			P	S	W
Double Chocolate	C	E			P	S	W

EDWARD & SONS:

Brown Rice Snaps:

	CORN	EGGS	MILK	NUTS	PEANUT	SOY	WHEAT
Buckwheat/No Salt							W
Buckwheat/Tamari						S	W
No Salt/Sesame							
Onion/Garlic							
Tamari/Seaweed						S	
Tamari/Sesame						S	
Crunchy Crackerballs					P	S	W

Miso-Cup Instant Soup Mix:

	CORN	EGGS	MILK	NUTS	PEANUT	SOY	WHEAT
Original						S	
Seaweed						S	

Miso Plus Dip Mix Ingredients:

	CORN	EGGS	MILK	NUTS	PEANUT	SOY	WHEAT
Chive						S	
Jalapeño						S	

Natural Temptations Candy:

	CORN	EGGS	MILK	NUTS	PEANUT	SOY	WHEAT
Cinnamon							
Peppermint							

Snack Sacks:

	CORN	EGGS	MILK	NUTS	PEANUT	SOY	WHEAT
Sea Vegie Chips	C						W
Vegie Chips	C						W

EGG ROLLS, frozen:

	CORN	EGGS	MILK	NUTS	PEANUT	SOY	WHEAT
(Empire Kosher) Miniature	C					S	W
(Health Valley Foods):							
Egg					P	S	W
Lobster					P	S	W
Shrimp					P	S	W
Teriyaki & Nut			M		P	S	W
(La Choy):							
Lobster	C	E	M		P	S	W

Food Item	C O R N	E G G S	M I L K	N U T S	P E A N U T	S O Y	W H E A T
Meat & Shrimp	C				P	S	W
Shrimp	C		M			S	W
EGG SUBSTITUTES:							
Egg Beaters (Fleischmann's):							
Regular	C	E					
With Cheez	C	E	M				
Egg Replacer (Ener-G Foods)							
EGGNOG:							
(Farm Best)	C	E	M				
(Flav-O-Rich)	C	E	M		P	S	
EGGPLANT, frozen (Mrs. Paul's):							
Eggplant Parmigiana	C		M		P	S	W
French Fried Eggplant Sticks	C		M		P	S	W
ENER-G FOODS:							
Baking Ingredients & Mixes (See also							
Wheat-Free Products below):							
Baking Powder							
Calcium Carbonate							
Calcium Chloride							
Corn Bran	C						
Corn Mix	C						
Egg Replacer							
Methylcellulose							
Potato Flour, fine							
Potato Mix							
Potato Starch							
Rice Baking Mix, brown	C			N			
Rice Baking Mix, white							
Rice Bran							
Rice Flour, brown							
Rice Flour, white							
Rice Mix							
Rice Mix, low sodium							
Rice Polish							
Rice Starch							
Soy-free Shortening							
Sweet Rice Flour							
Tapioca Flour							
Xanthan Gum	C						

Food Item	CORN	EGGS	MILK	NUTS	PEANUT	SOY	WHEAT
Bread:							
Brown Rice				N			
Rice & Fiber	C					S	
Rice & Starch	C		M			S	
White Rice							
Xanthan	C	E				S	
Yeast-Free Rice	C						
Bread Crumbs				N			
Buns & Rolls:							
Brown Rice Hamburger				N			
Rice Cinnamon Rolls	C					S	
White Rice Hamburger							
White Rice Hotdog							
Cake:							
Coffeecake:							
Apple-filled	C		M			S	
Raspberry-filled	C		M			S	
Fruitcake	C	E		N		S	
Cereal:							
Corn Germ Cereal	C						
Chocolate Crisps	C		M			S	
Cookies:							
Aglutella Vanilla-filled	C				P	S	
Chocolate Sandwich	C					S	
Date, no sugar added		E					
Dutch Cocoa	C					S	
Lemon Sandwich	C					S	
Lemon Shortbread	C					S	
Macaroons	C	E					
Orange	C					S	
Rice Carob	C	E				S	
Rice Chocolate	C	E			P	S	
Rice Peanut Butter	C	E	M		P	S	
Rice Spice	C	E				S	
Rice Walnut	C	E		N		S	
Crackers:							
Cinnamon Crackers	C					S	
Hol-Grain Gluten-free, Wheat-free							
Crackers:							
Salted							

Food Item	C O R N	E G G S	M I L K	N U T S	P E A N U T	S O Y	W H E A T
Unsalted							
Kitanihon Rice Crunch Crackers:							
Cheese	C		M		P	S	
Onion & Garlic						S	
Plain						S	
Melba Toast				N			
Croutons:							
Italian	C		M			S	
Plain	C					S	
Date Muffins							
Doughnuts:							
Apple Flavor	C		M			S	
Banana	C		M			S	
Banana, chocolate-iced	C		M			S	
Plain, chocolate-iced	C	E		N		S	
Plain Rice	C	E		N		S	
Pumpkin	C					S	
Pumpkin, chocolate-iced	C					S	
Med-Diet:							
Gluten-free, Wheat-free							
Instant Soups:							
Cream of Mushroom	C		M			S	
Tomato	C						
Seasonings:							
All-purpose	C						
All-purpose with Lemon	C						
Herb							
Salad	C		M				
Milk:							
Cultured Buttermilk			M				
NutQuik				N			
Pasta (See **PASTA**)							
Rice Pizza Shells	C					S	
SoyQuik						S	
Wheat-Free Products, with Gluten:							
Barley Mix							W
Millet							W
Oat Bran							W
Oat Mix							W
100% Rye Cereal							W

Food Item	CORN	EGGS	MILK	NUTS	PEANUT	SOY	WHEAT
Rice 'N Rye Bread Mix							W
ENTENMANN'S:							
All Butter Pound Loaf	C	E	M		P	S	W
Apple Puffs	C	E	M		P	S	W
Apple Raisin Coffee Cake	C	E	M	N	P	S	W
Apricot Danish Twist	C	E	M	N	P	S	W
Banana Crunch Cake	C	E	M		P	S	W
Bavarian Creme Coffee Cake	C	E	M		P	S	W
Blueberry Crumb Pie	C		M	N		S	W
Butter Sunshine	C	E	M		P	S	W
Cheese Coffee Cake	C	E	M		P	S	W
Cheese Topped Buns	C	E	M		P	S	W
Cherry Cheese Danish	C	E	M		P	S	W
Chocolate Chip Cookies	C	E				S	W
Chocolate Chip Crumb Loaf	C	E	M		P	S	W
Cinnamon Danish Twist	C	E	M	N	P	S	W
Country Style Donuts	C	E	M	N	P	S	W
Crumb Coffee Cake	C	E	M	N	P	S	W
Danish Coconut Tea Ring	C	E	M	N	P	S	W
Danish Ring (butter filling)	C	E	M		P	S	W
Devil's Food Crumb Donuts	C	E	M		P	S	W
Filled Chocolate Chip Crumb	C	E	M		P	S	W
Filled Donuts (Bavarian Creme)	C	E	M		P	S	W
Fruit and Fibre Muffins:							
Cinnamon Apple Raisin		E	M			S	W
Fruit Topped Buns, apple	C	E	M		P	S	W
Lemon Filled French Crumb	C	E	M	N	P	S	W
Lemon Pie	C	E	M			S	W
Marshmallow Iced Devil's Food	C	E	M		P	S	W
Old Fashioned Apple Strudel	C	E	M		P	S	W
Raisin Loaf	C	E	M		P	S	W
Rich Frosted Donuts	C	E	M		P	S	W
Sunshine Orange Danish Ring	C	E	M	N	P	S	W
EREWHON:							
Ready-to-eat-cereals:							
Crispy Brown Rice:							
Low sodium							W
Regular							W
Fruit 'n Wheat				N			W
Raisin Bran							W

Food Item	CORN	EGGS	MILK	NUTS	PEANUT	SOY	WHEAT
Wheat Flakes							W
Hot Cereals:							
Barley Plus							W
Brown Rice Cream							
Oat Bran with Wheat Germ							W
Granola:							
Date Nut	C			N			W
Honey Almond	C			N			W
Maple	C			N			W
Number Nine, with Bran, no salt	C			N			W
Spiced apple	C			N			W
Sunflower Crunch	C						W
Japanese Products:							
Crackers:							
Brown Rice							
Brown Rice, Shoyu						S	W
Koishi						S	W
Nori Maki						S	W
Misos:							
Genmai						S	
Hatcho						S	
Kome						S	
Mugi						S	W
Pastas:							
80% Buckwheat Soba							W
40% Buckwheat Soba							W
Ramen Dashi						S	W
Ramen Pasta							W
Udon							W
Shoyu Tamari						S	W
Sweets:							
Barley							W
Cinnamon							W
Ginger							W
Peppermint							W
Plum							W
Ume							W
Seed and Nut Butters							
Almond				N			
Cashew				N			

Food Item	CORN	EGGS	MILK	NUTS	PEANUT	SOY	WHEAT
Peanut, salted and unsalted:							
Chunky					P		
Creamy					P		
Sesame Butter							
Sesame Tahini							
Sunflower Butter							
Teas:							
Mu #9							
Mu #16							
EQUAL, sugar substitute:							
Packets	C						
Tablets	C		M				
EXTRACTS (See also **FLAVORS, ARTIFICIAL**):							
(French's):							
Almond	C			N			
Anise	C						
Brandy	C						
Lemon	C						
Orange	C						
Peppermint	C						
Rum	C						
Sherry	C						
Vanilla, pure	C						
Wintergreen	C						
Lemon (Spice Classics)	C						W
Orange (McCormick)	C						W
Vanilla (Spice Classics)	C						W
(Walnut Acres):							
Vanilla Extract	C						W

Food Item	C O R N	E G G S	M I L K	N U T S	P E A N U T	S O Y	W H E A T

F

FALAFEL MIX:
  (Fantastic) | | | | | | S | W
  (Near East) | | | | | | S | W

Food Item	C	E	M	N	P	S	W
FALAFEL MIX:							
(Fantastic)						S	W
(Near East)						S	W
FEARN NATURAL FOODS:							
Baking Mix:							
Brown Rice						S	
Rice						S	
Bread & Muffin Mix:							
Bran Muffin			M			S	W
Burger Mixes:							
Brazil Nut				N	P	S	W
Sesame						S	W
Sunflower					P	S	W
Corn Bread	C		M			S	W
Cake Mix:							
Banana Cake	C	E	M		P	S	W
Carob Cake	C	E	M		P	S	W
Carrot Cake	C	E	M		P	S	W
Spice Cake	C	E	M		P	S	W
Dry Mixes:							
Bean Barley Stew	C	E	M		P	S	W
Blackbean Creole Mix	C	E	M		P	S	
Breakfast Patty Mix						S	W
Falafel						S	
Tri-Bean Casserole	C	E	M		P	S	
Lecithin:							
Liquid						S	
Mint Flavored Liquid						S	
Naturfresh:							
Corn Germ	C						
Raw Wheat Germ							W
Non-Fat Dry Milk			M				
Pancake Mix:							
Buckwheat						S	W

Food Item	C O R N	E G G S	M I L K	N U T S	P E A N U T	S O Y	W H E A T
Rich Earth						S	W
7 Grain Buttermilk:							
Low-sodium	C		M			S	W
Regular	C		M			S	W W
Soy-O						S	W W
Whole Wheat						S	W
Rice Flour							
Soya Granules						S	
Soya Powder						S	
Soya Protein Isolate						S	
Soy-O Cereal						S	W
Soups, mixes:							
Lentil Minestrone	C	E	M		P	S	W
Split Pea	C	E	M		P	S	
FISH, frozen:							
(Gorton's):							
Light Recipe, Tempura Batter	C	E				S	W
(Health Valley Foods):							
Alaskan Fish:							
Fillets	C		M		P	S	W
Sticks	C		M		P	S	W
(Mrs. Paul's):							
Au Naturel:							
Haddock							W
Ocean Perch							W
Battered:							
Batter Dipped, Cod	C		M			S	W
Crunchy Light Batter:							
Fish	C	E	M			S	W
Flounder	C	E	M			S	W
Haddock	C	E	M			S	W
Supreme, Fish	C	E	M			S	W
Breaded, Crispy Crunchy:							
Flounder	C	E	M			S	W
Haddock	C	E	M			S	W
Ocean Perch	C	E	M			S	W
Breaded, Light:							
Fish	C	E	M			S	W
Flounder	C	E	M			S	W
Sole	C	E	M			S	W

Food Item	C O R N	E G G S	M I L K	N U T S	P E A N U T	S O Y	W H E A T
Buttered Fish Fillets			M				
Catfish Fillets	C	E	M			S	W
Catfish Fillet Strips	C	E	M			S	W
Fried:							
Clams	C		M			S	W
Combination Seafood	C	E	M		P	S	W
Scallops	C		M		P	S	W
Shrimp	C		M			S	W
(Van de Kamp's):							
Batter Dipped Fish Fillets	C	E	M			S	W
Today's Catch, Flounder							
FISH ENTRÉES, frozen:							
(Mrs. Paul's) *en Croute:*							
Crab Imperial	C	E	M			S	W
Fish Divan	C	E	M			S	W
Lobster Americaine	C	E	M			S	W
Salmon Veloute	C	E	M			S	W
Scallops St. Jacques	C	E	M			S	W
Seafood Newburg	C	E	M			S	W
(Mrs. Paul's) Light Seafood Entrée:							
Fillet of Flounder with Shrimp	C	E	M		P	S	W
Fillet of Sole with Shrimp	C	E	M		P	S	W
Fish & Pasta Florentine	C	E	M				W
Flounder Divan with Shrimp	C	E	M		P	S	W
Seafood Newburg	C	E	M			S	W
Shrimp Oriental	C				P	S	W
Shrimp Primavera	C	E	M			S	W
Sole Divan with Shrimp	C	E	M		P	S	W
FISH CAKES:							
(Mrs. Paul's):							
Fish Cakes	C	E	M		P	S	W
Fish Cake Thins	C	E	M			S	W
FISH, GEFILTE (See **GEFILTE FISH**)							
FISH STICKS:							
(Mrs. Paul's):							
Crispy Crunchy	C	E	M			S	W
Crunchy Light Batter	C	E	M			S	W
Crunchy, with Minced Fish	C	E	M			S	W
FLA-VOR-AID (See **DRINK MIX**)							

Food Item	CORN	EGGS	MILK	NUTS	PEANUT	SOY	WHEAT
FLA-VOR-ICE							
(See **FROZEN DESSERTS**)							
FLAVORS, ARTIFICIAL							
(See also **EXTRACTS**):							
(French's):							
Banana	C						
Black Walnut	C			N			
Butter	C		M				
Cherry	C						
Chocolate	C						
Coconut	C						
Maple	C						
Peach	C						
Pineapple	C						
Pistachio	C			N			
Raspberry	C						
Strawberry	C						
Vanilla, imitation	C						
FRANKFURTERS (See also							
KNOCKWURST, SAUSAGE):							
Beef:							
(Health Valley Foods):							
Beef Wieners							
(Hormel):							
Beef Wieners	C						
(Hygrade's):							
Ball Park	C						
Beef	C						
(Nathan's) Skinless	C					S	W
(Oscar Mayer)	C						
Beef, Kosher:							
(Shofar)	C						
Chicken:							
(Health Valley Foods):							
Chicken Wieners							
(Hygrade's) *Grillmaster*	C						
Meat:							
(Hormel) Meat Wieners	C						
(Oscar Mayer):							
Hot Dogs:							

Food Item	CORN	EGGS	MILK	NUTS	PEANUT	SOY	WHEAT
Bacon & Cheddar Cheese	C		M				
Cheese	C		M				
Nacho Cheese	C		M				
Little Wieners	C						
Wieners	C						
Turkey:							
(Health Valley Foods):							
Turkey Wieners							
(Louis Rich):							
Turkey Franks	C						
Turkey Cheese Franks	C		M				
Turkey Smoked Sausage	C						
Mr. Turkey (Bil Mar):							
Cheese Franks	C		M				
Franks	C						

FRANKFURTERS, SMOKED
(See **SMOKED FRANKFURTERS**)
FREIHOFER'S (See **CAKE, COOKIES, MUFFINS**)
FRIJOLES:
(Fantastic) mix
FRITTERS, frozen (Mrs. Paul's):

Food Item	CORN	EGGS	MILK	NUTS	PEANUT	SOY	WHEAT
Apple	C		M		P	S	W
Corn	C	E	M			S	W

FROSTING:
Chocolate:

Food Item	CORN	EGGS	MILK	NUTS	PEANUT	SOY	WHEAT
(Duncan Hines)	C				P	S	W

Chocolate Chocolate Chip:

Food Item	CORN	EGGS	MILK	NUTS	PEANUT	SOY	WHEAT
(Betty Crocker)	C		M		P	S	W

Fudge:

Food Item	CORN	EGGS	MILK	NUTS	PEANUT	SOY	WHEAT
(Duncan Hines) Dark Dutch	C				P	S	W
(Pillsbury) Chocolate Fudge	C	E			P	S	

Milk Chocolate:

Food Item	CORN	EGGS	MILK	NUTS	PEANUT	SOY	WHEAT
(Duncan Hines)	C		M		P	S	W

Vanilla:

Food Item	CORN	EGGS	MILK	NUTS	PEANUT	SOY	WHEAT
(Duncan Hines)	C		M		P	S	W
(Pillsbury)	C	E			P	S	

(Wilton):

Food Item	CORN	EGGS	MILK	NUTS	PEANUT	SOY	WHEAT
Chocolate Buttercream	C		M		P	S	W
Vanilla Butter	C		M		P	S	W

Food Item	C O R N	E G G S	M I L K	N U T S	P E A N U T	S O Y	W H E A T
FROSTING MIX/ICING MIX:							
Artificially Sweetened:							
(Sweet 'n Low):							
Chocolate	C		M		P	S	W
White	C		M		P	S	W
FROZEN DESSERTS &							
CONFECTIONS:							
Dole Whip:							
Banana	C	E	M		P	S	W
Lime	C	E	M		P	S	
Orange	C	E	M		P	S	
Pineapple	C	E	M		P	S	
Strawberry	C	E	M		P	S	
Fla-vor-ice:							
Grape	C						W
Lemon-Lime	C						W
Orange	C						W
Strawberry	C						W
Fruit & Cream Bars (Dole)	C		M				
Fruit Juicee (Minute Maid) cherry	C						
Fruit 'N Juice Bars (Dole)	C						
Fruit Sorbet (Dole), all flavors	C						
Fudge Bars, frozen:							
(Flav-O-Rich)	C		M				
Fudgsicle (Popsicle):	C		M		P	S	W
Pop-ice:							
Grape	C						W
Lemon-Lime	C						W
Orange	C						W
Strawberry	C						W
Pudding Pops (Jell-O):							
Vanilla	C		M	P		S	W
Chocolate-Vanilla Swirl	C		M		P	S	W
FROZFRUIT:							
Banana	C		M				
Cantaloupe	C						
Cherry	C						
Coconut	C		M				
Lemon	C						
Lime	C						

Food Item	C O R N	E G G S	M I L K	N U T S	P E A N U T	S O Y	W H E A T
Mango	C						
Orange	C						
Peach	C						
Pineapple	C						
Raspberry, milk base	C		M				
Raspberry, water base	C						
Strawberry, milk base	C		M				
Strawberry, water base	C						
Watermelon	C						
FRUIT AND CREAM BARS (Dole)	C		M				
FRUIT BARS (Fruit Corners), cherry	C					S	W

FRUIT, BRANDIED:
  (Raffetto):
    Apricots
    Bing Cherries
    Cherries Jubilee
    Figs
    Fruits
    Peach Halves
    Peaches
    Pears
FRUIT, CANNED:
  Fruit Cocktail:
    (Libby's), *Lite*
  Mixed:
    (Del Monte):

Chunky, heavy syrup	C						

      Chunky, *Lite*
      Fruit Cup (Del Monte), Lite
  Peaches:
    (Del Monte) *Lite* Peaches
    (Libby's) *Lite*
  Pineapple:
    (Dole) unsweetened:
      Chunks
      Slices
    (Premier Japan):
      Umeboshi (plums)
FRUIT DRINKS, asceptically packed:

Food Item	C O R N	E G G S	M I L K	N U T S	P E A N U T	S O Y	W H E A T
Lemonade:							
Koolers (*Kool-Aid*)	C						
FRUIT DRINKS, bottled:							
(Veryfine):							
Fruit Punch	C				P	S	
Grape Drink	C						
(Welch's):							
Grape Juice Beverage	C						
Welchade Grape Drink	C						
FRUIT DRINKS, dairy pack:							
(Flav-O-Rich):							
Orange Joy	C						
Dair-E Lemonade							
Five Percent Fruit Drinks:							
Fruit Punch	C				P	S	
Lemon-Lime	C				P	S	
Strawberry	C						W
Fruit Punch:							
(Minute Maid)	C						
(Tropicana)	C				P	S	W
Grapeade (Minute Maid)	C						
Lemonade:							
(Minute Maid)	C						
(Tropicana)	C						
(Tropicana):							
Apple Drink	C		M				W
Fruit Punch	C				P	S	W
Grape Drink	C						
Orange-Pineapple	C				P	S	W
FRUIT, FROZEN:							
(Birds Eye):							
Mixed Fruit, Lite Syrup	C						
Strawberries, Lite Syrup							
FRUIT JUICE (See also **JUICE,** fruit name or brand name)							
(Tropicana):							
Apple Juice							
Grapefruit Juice							

Food Item	C O R N	E G G S	M I L K	N U T S	P E A N U T	S O Y	W H E A T
Orange Juice:							
Home Style							
Pure Premium							
Tropicana							
Orange-Pineapple							
(Welch's):							
Orchard Apple-Grape							
Orchard Harvest Blend							
Orchard North Country Blend							
Orchard Vineyard Blend							
Purple Grape	C						
Red Grape	C						
Sparkling Red Grape							
Sparkling White Grape							
Tomato							
White Grape	C						
FRUIT JUICE, FROZEN:							
(Welch's):							
Cranberry-Apple Juice Cocktail	C						
Cranberry-Grape Juice Cocktail	C						
Cranberry Juice Cocktail	C						
Orchard Apple-Grape							
Orchard Grape Juice							
Orchard Harvest Blend							
Orchard North Country Blend							
Sweetened Grape Juice	C						
FRUIT JUICEE (Minute Maid) cherry	C						
FRUIT 'N JUICE BARS (Dole)	C						
FRUIT 'N SAUCE (Lucky Leaf):							
Apple Apricot	C						
Apple Cherry	C						
Apple Peach	C						
FRUIT, PRESERVED:							
(Raffetto):							
Assorted Fruits							
Harlequin Oranges							
Orange Slices							
Peaches in *Giroux* Grenadine	C						
Pickled Peaches	C						W
Pineapple Sticks							

Food Item	CORN	EGGS	MILK	NUTS	PEANUT	SOY	WHEAT
Premium Kumquats							
Purple Plums in Sherry							
FRUIT ROLL UPS:							
(Fruit Corners):							
Apricot	C				P	S	W
Orange	C				P	S	W W
Raspberry	C				P	S	W
(Sunkist):							
Cherry	C						
Strawberry	C						
FRUIT SNACKS (See brand names)							
FRUIT SORBET (Dole)	C						
FRUIT SPREADS (See also							
JAM/JELLY):							
(Poiret):							
Pear & Apple							
Pear & Apricot							
Pear & Black Cherry							
Pear & Lemon							
Pear & Orange							
Pear & Passion Fruit							
Pear & Raspberry							
Pear & Strawberry							
FRUIT SWIRL BARS (Fruit Corners):							
Real Raspberries & Cream	C	E	M		P	S	W
Real Strawberries & Cream	C	E	M		P	S	W
FUDGE BARS, frozen:							
(Flav-O-Rich)	C		M				
Fudgsicle (Popsicle):	C		M		P	S	W
FUN FRUITS (Sunkist):							
Cherry	C	E			P	S	W

Food Item	CORN	EGGS	MILK	NUTS	PEANUT	SOY	WHEAT

G

Food Item	CORN	EGGS	MILK	NUTS	PEANUT	SOY	WHEAT
GATORADE, lemon-lime	C				P	S	
GELATIN:							
Royal (Nabisco), regular:							
Apple							
Blackberry							
Cherry							
Lemon							
Lemon-Lime							
Lime							
Orange							
Peach							
Pineapple							
Raspberry							
Strawberry							
Strawberry Banana							
Tropical Fruit							
Royal (Nabisco) sugar-free:							
Cherry							
Lime							
Orange							
Raspberry							
Strawberry							
(Walnut Acres), regular							
GERBER (See **BABY FOOD**)							
GEFILTE FISH:							
(Manischewitz), unsalted		E					W
GRAHAM CRACKER CRUMBS:							
(Sunshine)	C		M		P	S	W
GRAHAM CRACKERS							
(See **CRACKERS**)							
GINGER:							
Pickled (Premier Japan)							
Stem Ginger in Syrup (Raffetto)	C						
GRAIN MIXES:							

Food Item	CORN	EGGS	MILK	NUTS	PEANUT	SOY	WHEAT
(Walnut Acres):							
Amaranth Medley							W
Near East Kasha							W
Savory Millet						S	W
Sustains							W
GRANOLA (See **CEREAL**)							
GRANOLA BARS:							
Granola *Dipps* (Quaker):							
Caramel Nut	C	E	M	N	P	S	W
Chocolate Chip	C	E	M	N	P	S	W
Mint Chocolate Chip	C	E	M	N	P	S	W
Peanut Butter	C	E	M	N	P	S	W
Raisin & Almond	C	E	M	N	P	S	W
Rocky Road	C	E	M	N	P	S	
New Trail (Hershey's):							
Peanut Butter	C		M		P	S	W
Peanut Butter & Chocolate Chip	C		M		P	S	W
GRANOLA SNACKS:							
Kudos (Mars):							
Chocolate Chip	C	E	M	N	P	S	W
Nutty Fudge	C	E	M	N	P	S	W
Peanut Butter	C	E	M	N	P	S	W
GRAPEFRUIT JUICE:							
Bottled (Ocean Spray)							
Dairy Pak (Minute Maid)							
GRAVY, CANNED:							
(Franco-American):							
Au Jus	C		M			S	W
Chicken	C		M			S	W
Turkey	C		M			S	W
GRAVY MIXES:							
(French's):							
Au Jus	C		M				W
Brown	C		M				W
Gravy for Chicken	C		M				
Gravy for Pork	C		M				W
Gravy for Turkey	C		M				W
Mushroom	C		M				W
Onion	C		M				W
GRAVY MASTER	C					S	W

Food Item	CORN	EGGS	MILK	NUTS	PEANUT	SOY	WHEAT
GRENADINE:							
(Giroux)	C						
GUACAMOLE MIX:							
(Concord)	C		M				W
GUM:							
(*Beech-Nut*):							
Cinnamon	C					S	
Fancy Fruit	C					S	
Peppermint	C					S	
Spearmint	C					S	
Bubble Yum, regular:							
Bananaberry Split	C						
Cherry	C					S	
Fruit	C					S	
Grape	C					S	
Luscious Lime	C					S	
Pink Lemonade	C					S	
Spearmint	C						
Strawberry	C						
Tropical Punch	C						
Wacky Fruit	C					S	
Bubble Yum, sugarless:							
Fruit	C					S	
Grape	C					S	
Orange	C					S	
Strawberry	C						
Candy Coated (*Beechies*):							
Fruit	C					S	
Peppermint	C					S	
Pepsin	C					S	
Spearmint	C					S	
Care-Free, sugarless, regular:							
Cinnamon	C						
Fruit	C						
Peppermint	C						
Spearmint	C						
Care-Free, sugarless, bubble gum:							
Fruit	C						
Orange	C						
Strawberry	C						

Food Item	CORN	EGGS	MILK	NUTS	PEANUT	SOY	WHEAT
Wintergreen	C						
Fruit Stripe, regular:							
Cherry						S	
Lemon						S	
Lime						S	
Orange						S	
Fruit Stripe, bubble gum:							
Cherry						S	
Fruit						S	
Grape						S	
Lemon						S	
Replay:							
Cinnamon						S	
Peppermint						S	
Spearmint						S	

Food Item	C O R N	E G G S	M I L K	N U T S	P E A N U T	S O Y	W H E A T

H

HALVAH:
  (Fantastic Foods):
    Carob-Sesame | C | E | | N | P | S | |
    Cashew-Currant | C | E | | N | P | S | |
    Sesame-Honey | C | E | | N | P | S | |
HAM:
  (Hormel):
    Black Label Canned Ham | | E | M | | | S | |
    Bone-In | C | E | | | | | |
    Boneless Buffet | | | M | | | S | W |
    Cure 81 | | | | | | | |
    Curemaster | | | | | | | |
    Ham Patties | | E | | | | | |
    Ham Roll | | | | | | | |
  (Oscar Mayer):
    Boneless Jubilee | | | | | | | |
    Jubilee, canned | | | | | | | |
    Jubilee, slice | | | | | | | |
    Jubilee, steaks | | | | | | | |
HAM, chopped & canned:
  (Hormel) Chunk | | | M | | | | |
HAM, deviled:
  (Hormel) | C | | | | | S | |
  (Underwood) | | | | | | | |
HAM ENTRÉES, frozen:
  Ham Steak (*Le Menu*) | C | | M | | P | S | W |
HARDEE'S:
  Breads:
    Biscuit | | | M | | | S | W |
    Bun | C | | | | P | S | W |
  Condiments:
    Mayonnaise | C | E | | | | S | W |
    Mustard | C | | | | | | W |
    Tartar Sauce | C | E | | | | S | W |

Food Item	CORN	EGGS	MILK	NUTS	PEANUT	SOY	WHEAT
Meat, Fish, Poultry:							
Chicken Fillet	C	E	M			S	W
Fish Fillet	C					S	W
Hot Dog	C						
Sausage	C					S	W
Toppings:							
American Cheese	C	E	M		P	S	
Chili	C		M			S	W
HAWAIIAN PUNCH (See also							
DRINK MIX):							
Lite	C						W
HEALTH VALLEY FOODS:							
Baked Beans, canned:							
Boston-Style							
Vegetarian with Miso						S	W
Cereals:							
Amaranth:							
Regular:	C						W
With Bananas	C			N			W
With Raisins	C						W
Baby Cereal:							
Instant Brown Rice							W
Sprouted Cereal with Bananas							W
Bran:							
Regular:							W
With Apples, Cinnamon							W
With Bananas							W
With Hawaiian Fruit							W
With Raisins							W
Granola (*Real*):							
Almond Crunch				N		S	W
Apple Cinnamon				N		S	W
Hawaiian Fruit				N		S	W
Maple Nut				N		S	W
Raisin Nut				N		S	W
Healthy Crunch:							
Almond Date				N		S	W
Apple Cinnamon						S	W
Hawaiian Fruit				N		S	W
Hearts O' Bran:							
Apples & Cinnamon							W

Food Item	CORN	EGGS	MILK	NUTS	PEANUT	SOY	WHEAT
Raisins & Spice							W
Lites:							
Brown Rice							
Golden Corn	C						
Golden Wheat							W
Miller's Bran Flakes							W
Orangeola:							
Regular:						S	W
With Almonds, Dates				N		S	W
With Bananas, Coconut, & Hawaiian Fruit						S	W
Sprouts 7:							
With Bananas, Hawaiian Fruit							W
With Raisins							W
Stoned Wheat:							
Flakes							W
Raisin Bran Flakes							W
Wheat Germ:							
Regular							W
With Almonds, Dates				N			W
With Bananas, Hawaiian Fruit							W
Chili:							
Con Carne						S	W
Vegetarian with Beans:							
Mild						S	W
Mild, no salt						S	
Spicy						S	W
Spicy, no salt						S	
With Lentils						S	
Condiments:							
Catch-Up:							
No-salt							
Regular							
Mayonnaise	C	E				S	W
Mustard	C						W
Cookies:							
Date Pecan			M	N			W
Honey Jumbos:							
Cinnamon	C	E	M		P	S	W
Oatmeal			M			S	W

Food Item	CORN	EGGS	MILK	NUTS	PEANUT	SOY	WHEAT
Peanut Butter	C	E	M		P	S	W
Oatmeal			M				W
Peanut Butter			M		P		W
Raisin Bran			M				W
Snaps:							
Animal			M			S	W
Carob			M				W
Cinnamon			M			S	W
Coconut			M				W
Ginger			M				W
Honey			M			S	W
Lemon			M				W
Yogurt			M				W
Crackers:							
Amaranth	C	E			P	S	W
Cheese Wheels			M				W
Herb	C						W
Honey Graham	C	E	M		P	S	W
Sesame	C						W
7-Grain, 7-Vegetable	C						W
Stoned Wheat	C						W
Wheat & Sweet Rye	C						W
Yogurt & Green Onion	C		M				W
Frozen Foods:							
Alaskan Fish:							
Fillets	C		M		P	S	W
Sticks	C		M		P	S	W
Chinese Rolls:							
Egg					P	S	W
Lobster					P	S	W
Shrimp					P	S	W
Teriyaki & Nut			M		P	S	W
Lean Living Dinners:							
Cheese Enchiladas	C		M			S	
Chicken à la King		E	M				W
Chicken Crepes		E	M				W
Spinach Lasagna			M				W
Spinach-Mushroom Casserole		E	M				W
Meals For Two:							
Cheddar Chicken			M			S	W

Food Item	CORN	EGGS	MILK	NUTS	PEANUT	SOY	WHEAT
Cheese Eggplant			M			S	W
Cheese Enchiladas	C		M			S	W
Spinach Lasagna			M			S	W
Stuffed Peppers			M			S	W
Tortillas, *Corntillas*	C						
Fruit Bakes:							
Apple				N		S	W
Date				N		S	W
Raisin				N		S	W
Luncheon Meats:							
Beef:							
Bologna							
Knockwurst							
Salami							
Wieners							
Chicken:							
Bologna							
Wieners							
Turkey Wieners							
Oils:							
Best Blend	C					S	
Corn	C						
Olive							
Peanut					P		
Safflower							
Sesame							
Soy						S	
Sunflower							
Pancake Mix:							
Original Recipe							W
With Buttermilk			M				W
Pasta:							
Amaranth, spaghetti							W
Regular:							
Elbows	C						W
Lasagna	C						W
Spaghetti	C						W
With 4 Vegetables, elbows	C						W
With Spinach:							
Lasagna	C						W

Food Item	CORN	EGGS	MILK	NUTS	PEANUT	SOY	WHEAT
Spaghetti	C						W
Peanut Butter, all varieties					P		
Potato Chips:							
Regular							
Country Chips							
Country Ripples							
No Salt, all varieties							
Pretzels:							
Natural	C						W
Whole Wheat	C						W
Salad Dressings & Dips:							
Avocado	C	E	M		P	S	
Blue Cheese	C	E	M		P	S	
Creamy Yogurt	C	E	M		P	S	
Green Goddess	C	E	M		P	S	
No-Salt:							
Avocado	C	E	M		P	S	
Original Herb	C	E	M		P	S	
1000 Island	C	E	M		P	S	
Original Herb	C	E	M		P	S	
Real French						S	
Real Cheese & Herbs			M			S	
Real Italian						S	
Roquefort	C	E	M		P	S	
1000 Island	C	E	M		P	S	
Seasonings, *Instead of Salt:*							
All Purpose							
Chicken							
Fish							
Steak & Hamburgers							
Vegetables							
Snacks:							
Buenitos:							
Nacho Cheese & Chili	C		M				
Regular	C						
Unsalted	C						
Cheddar Lites:							
Regular	C		M				
Unsalted	C		M				

Food Item	CORN	EGGS	MILK	NUTS	PEANUT	SOY	WHEAT
Corn Chips:							
Regular	C						
Unsalted	C						
With Cheese	C		M				
Yogurt	C		M				
Tortilla Strips:							
Regular	C						
Cheese	C		M				
12 Vegetable	C						
Yogurt & Green Onion	C		M				
Soda:							
Apple	C						
Cola	C						
Ginger Ale	C						
Ginseng Root Beer	C						
Grape	C						
Lemon-Lime	C						
Mandarin-Lime	C						
Root Beer	C						
Sarsaparilla	C						
Wild Berry	C						
Soup, Canned:							
Vegetable Beef	C						W
Vegetable Chicken	C						W
Soy Products:							
Soy Moo, beverage:							
Carob						S	
Plain						S	
Tamari-ya soy sauce						S	
Tofu-Ya tofu						S	
Tea:							
Lively Daytime							
Tranquil Evening							
Zesty Morning							
Tomato Sauce:							
No-Salt							
Pasta Sauce, *Bellissimo*			M				
Regular						S	W
Tuna:							
Chunk Light	C					S	

Food Item	CORN	EGGS	MILK	NUTS	PEANUT	SOY	WHEAT
No Salt	C					S	
HILLSHIRE FARM:							
Cheddarwurst	C		M			S	W
Hot Links:							
Beef	C						
Regular	C						
Knockwurst	C						
Polish Sausage	C					S	W
Polska Kielbasa:							
Beef	C					S	W
Mild	C					S	W
Regular	C					S	W
Smoked Sausage:							
Beef	C					S	W
Hot	C						
Original	C					S	W
HORMEL:							
Bacon:							
Black Label							
Canadian-style			M			S	W
Old Smokehouse			M			S	W
(Range)							
Red Label			M				
Salt Pork			M				
Bacon Bits			M			S	W
Canned Meats/Poultry:							
Chicken Vienna Sausage	C		M			S	W
Chunk:							
Breast of Chicken			M				
Ham			M				
Turkey			M				
White and Dark Chicken			M				
Creamed Dried Beef	C		M			S	W
Deviled Ham	C					S	
Deviled *Spam*						S	W
Spam							
Spam, smoke flavored	C						W
Spam with Cheese Chunks			M				
Pickled Pigs' Feet		E	M			S	W
Potted Meat Food Product			M			S	

Food Item	CORN	EGGS	MILK	NUTS	PEANUT	SOY	WHEAT
Vienna Sausage	C		M				
Canned Side Dishes/Entrées:							
Au Gratin Potatoes & Bacon	C		M			S	W
Beans & Bacon	C					S	W
Beans & Ham	C					S	W
Beans & Wieners	C					S	W
Beef Goulash	C		M			S	W
Beef Tamales	C		M			S	
Chili, Hot, with Beans	C					S	W
Chili Mac	C		M			S	W
Chili, No Beans	C					S	W
Chili with Beans	C					S	
Lasagna	C		M			S	W
Macaroni & Cheese	C		M			S	W
Noodles & Beef	C		M			S	W
Pork Chow Mein	C					S	W
Scalloped Potatoes & Ham	C		M			S	W
Sloppy Joes	C					S	W
Spaghetti & Beef	C		M			S	W
Spaghetti & Meatballs	C		M			S	W
Dinty Moore:							
Brunswick Stew	C		M			S	W
Beef Stew	C					S	
Hashed Potatoes & Beef						S	W
Noodles & Chicken	C		M			S	W
Dry Sausage:							
Pepperoni:							
Chunk Pepperoni			M				
Pepperoni		E	M				
Rosa Pepperoni			M				W
Rosa Grande Pepperoni			M			S	W
Sliced Pepperoni			M				
Prosciutto Ham			M			S	W
Salami:							
Chunk Hard Salami			M				
Cotto Salami			M			S	W
Hard Salami			M				
Piccolo Salami			M			S	W
Sliced Genoa Salami			M				
Sliced Hard Salami			M				

Food Item	C O R N	E G G S	M I L K	N U T S	P E A N U T	S O Y	W H E A T
Sliced Party Salami			M				
Soppresata Salami			M			S	W
Summer Sausage:							
Beefy Summer Sausage			M				
Lumberjack Beef Summer Sausage			M				W
Sliced Beef Summer Sausage			M				
Tangy Summer Sausage			M				
Thuringer:							
Old Smokehouse Thuringer			M				
Sliced Buffet Thuringer			M			S	W
Sliced *Old Smokehouse* Thuringer			M				
Viking Cervelat			M				
Ham:							
Black Label Canned Ham		E	M			S	
Bone-In	C	E					
Boneless Buffet			M			S	W
Cure 81							
Curemaster							
Ham Patties		E					
Ham Roll							
Mary Kitchen:							
Corned Beef Hash						S	
Roast Beef Hash						S	W
Perma-Fresh Lunch Meats:							
BBQ Loaf	C		M			S	
Beef Bologna	C						
Black Peppered Ham							
Bologna	C						W
Breast of Turkey	C		M			S	W
Buffet Loaf	C		M			S	W
Chopped Ham							
Cooked Ham	C		M				
Cotto Salami	C		M			S	
Genoa Salami	C		M				
Ham & Cheese Loaf	C		M			S	
Hard Salami			M				
Honey Loaf			M			S	W
(Iowa) Loaf			M			S	W
(Milwaukee) Smoky Thuringer		E	M			S	W
(New England) Luncheon Meat	C						

Food Item	CORN	EGGS	MILK	NUTS	PEANUT	SOY	WHEAT
Olive Loaf	C		M			S	
Pickle Loaf	C		M			S	
Smoked Cooked Ham						S	W
Spiced Luncheon Meat	C		M			S	
Prepared Sausage:							
Bologna:							
Coarse Ground Beef Bologna	C		M			S	W
Coarse Ground Bologna	C		M			S	
Fine Ground Bologna	C		M			S	
Braunschweiger	C		M				
Frankfurters and Wieners:							
Beef Wieners	C						
Meat Wieners	C						
Polish Sausage/Kielbasa:							
Kolbase Polish Sausage	C						
Polish Sausage	C		M			S	W
Skinless Kielbasa Polish Sausage	C		M			S	W
Sausage:							
Brown 'n Serve Sausage							
Midget Links, Pork Sausage							
Smoked Frankfurters and Sausage:							
Beef Wranglers Smoked Franks	C						
Skinless Smoked Sausage			M			S	
Smoked Pork Sausage (no link)							
Smokies:							
Cheezers Smoked Sausage	C		M				
Smoked Sausage	C						W
Wranglers (Range) Smoked							
Franks	C						
HORSERADISH:							
(Gold's):							
Home Style	C						W
Hot, Cream Style	C						W
(Premier Japan):							
Wasabi Powder (horseradish)							
HOT POCKETS:							
Ham 'N Cheese	C	E	M		P	S	W

Food Item	CORN	EGGS	MILK	NUTS	PEANUT	SOY	WHEAT

I

ICE CREAM (See also ICE CREAM NOVELTIES, FROZEN DESSERTS & CONFECTIONS)

(Baskin-Robbins):

Food Item	CORN	EGGS	MILK	NUTS	PEANUT	SOY	WHEAT
Bittersweet Chocolate Chip	C	E	M		P	S	
Black Walnut	C		M	N			W
Vanilla	C		M				W
(Ben & Jerry's):							
Butter Pecan		E	M	N			
Chocolate		E	M				
Coffee Heath Bar Crunch	C	E	M	N	P	S	
Dastardly Mash	C	E	M	N	P	S	
French Vanilla		E	M				
Fresh Georgia Peach		E	M				
Heathbar Crunch	C	E	M	N	P	S	
Mint with Oreo Cookies	C	E	M		P	S	W
Vanilla Chocolate Chunk		E	M				
White Russian		E	M				
(Dairy Charm):							
Black Walnut	C		M	N	P	S	W
Chocolate	C		M		P	S	
Chocolate Ripple	C		M		P	S	
Fudge Ripple	C		M		P	S	
Neopolitan	C		M		P	S	
Strawberry	C		M		P	S	
Vanilla	C		M		P	S	
(Dixieland):							
Black Walnut	C		M	N	P	S	W
Chocolate	C		M		P	S	
Chocolate Ripple	C		M		P	S	
Fudge Ripple	C		M		P	S	
Neopolitan	C		M		P	S	
Strawberry	C		M		P	S	
Vanilla	C		M		P	S	
(Dolly Madison):							

Food Item	CORN	EGGS	MILK	NUTS	PEANUT	SOY	WHEAT
Vanilla Chocolate Fudge	C		M		P	S	
(Flav-O-Rich):							
Banana Berry	C		M		P	S	W
Black Cherry	C		M		P	S	
Black Walnut	C		M	N	P	S	W
Butter Almond	C		M	N	P	S	
Butter Pecan	C		M	N	P	S	W
Cherry Vanilla	C		M		P	S	
Chocolate	C		M		P	S	
Chocolate Chip	C		M		P	S	W
Coffee	C		M		P	S	W
Cookies & Cream	C	E	M		P	S	W
Egg Nog	C	E	M		P	S	
Heavenly Hash	C	E	M	N	P	S	
Neopolitan	C		M		P	S	W
Peanut Butter 'N Fudge	C	E	M		P	S	W
Peach	C		M		P	S	
Piña Colada	C		M		P	S	
Rocky Road	C		M	N	P	S	W
Rum Raisin	C		M		P	S	W
Spumoni	C		M	N	P	S	
Strawberry	C		M		P	S	
Strawberry Cobbler	C	E	M		P	S	W
Vanilla	C		M		P	S	
Vanilla Slices	C		M		P	S	
(Frusen Glädjé):							
Chocolate Chocolate Chip		E	M				
Mocha Chip		E	M				
Vanilla		E	M				
(Häagen-Dazs):							
Coffee		E	M				
Honey Vanilla		E	M				
Sorbet & Cream:							
Orange & Cream	C	E	M				
Raspberry & Cream	C	E	M				
Vanilla		E	M				
(Louis Sherry):							
Strawberries 'n Cream	C		M				
(Pepperidge Farm):							
Chocolate Chocolate Chip	C	E	M		P	S	

Food Item	CORN	EGGS	MILK	NUTS	PEANUT	SOY	WHEAT
(Rich & Creamy):							
Butter Pecan	C	E	M	N	P	S	
Cherry Vanilla	C	E	M		P	S	W
Chocolate	C	E	M		P	S	
Chocolate Chip	C	E	M		P	S	
Coconut Cream	C	E	M		P	S	
Columbian Coffee	C	E	M		P	S	W
Cookies & Cream	C	E	M		P	S	W
French Vanilla	C	E	M				
German Chocolate	C	E	M	N	P	S	
Mint Chocolate Chip	C		M				W
Old Fashioned Vanilla	C	E	M		P	S	
Peach	C	E	M		P	S	
Pralines & Cream	C	E	M	N	P	S	
Real Strawberry	C	E	M		P	S	
Strawberry Cheesecake	C	E	M		P	S	
Vanilla Fudge	C	E	M		P	S	
Vanilla Swiss Chocolate Almond	C	E	M	N	P	S	
(Schrafft's), Chocolate	C	E	M		P	S	
(Steve's):							
Smores	C	E	M		P	S	W
Vanilla Super Chocolate Chunk	C	E	M		P	S	
(Tuscan Supreme):							
Rocky Road	C	E	M	N	P	S	
Vanilla	C	E	M		P	S	
(Welsh Farms):							
Coffee Royale	C		M		P	S	
Mint Chocolate Chip	C		M		P	S	
ICE CREAM, dietetic:							
(Estee) Vanilla	C		M		P	S	
(Flav-O-Rich):							
Chocolate	C		M		P	S	
Vanilla	C		M		P	S	
ICE CREAM MIX:							
(Salada):							
Peach	C		M		P	S	
Vanilla	C		M		P	S	
Wild Strawberry	C		M		P	S	
ICE CREAM NOVELTIES:							
Bars, chocolate-coated, vanilla:							

Food Item	CORN	EGGS	MILK	NUTS	PEANUT	SOY	WHEAT
(Borden)	C	E	M		P	S	
(Dolly Madison)	C	E	M		P	S	
(Flav-O-Rich)	C	E	M		P	S	
(Häagen-Dazs)	C	E	M		P	S	
Klondikes	C	E	M		P	S	
(Rich & Creamy)	C	E	M		P	S	W
Whammy (Good Humor)	C		M		P	S	
Bon Bons (Carnation)	C	E	M		P	S	W
Cake Roll (Green's)	C	E	M		P	S	W
Cream Bar, orange-coated ice cream:							
(Dolly Madison)	C		M		P	S	
Orange Cream (Flav-O-Rich)	C		M		P	S	W
Creamsicle	C		M		P	S	
Dream Bars (Flav-O-Rich)	C		M		P	S	
(Flav-O-Rich):							
Chocolate Peanut Cluster	C		M		P	S	
Drumsticks	C	E	M		P	S	W
Moon Pie	C	E	M		P	S	W
Tin Roof Sundae	C	E	M		P	S	W
(Good Humor):							
Strawberry Shortcake bar	C	E	M		P	S	W
Whammy:							
Chocolate	C		M		P	S	
Strawberry	C		M		P	S	
Vanilla	C		M		P	S	
(Häagen-Dazs):							
Bar, vanilla, chocolate coated	C	E	M		P	S	
Heaven bars (Carnation):							
Very Vanilla	C	E	M		P	S	W
Nestlé Crunch Bar (Flav-O-Rich)	C	E	M		P	S	W
Oreo Sandwiches	C	E	M		P	S	W
Sandwiches, vanilla:							
(Flav-O-Rich)	C	E	M		P	S	W
Orbit 5 (Flav-O-Rich)	C	E	M		P	S	W
Toffee:							
Bars (Heath)	C	E	M	N	P	S	
Sandwiches (Heath)	C	E	M	N	P	S	W
ICE MILK:							
Chocolate (Rich & Creamy)	C		M		P	S	
Chocolate Swirl (Farm Best)	C		M		P	S	W

Food Item	C O R N	E G G S	M I L K	N U T S	P E A N U T	S O Y	W H E A T
Fudge Twirl (Flav-O-Rich)	C		M		P	S	W
Strawberry Swirl (Farm Best)	C		M		P	S	W
Vanilla (Rich & Creamy)	C		M		P	S	
ICE POPS:							
(Dolly Madison):							
Cherry	C						
Fruit	C						
Orange	C						
(Flav-O-Rich)	C						
Life Savers (Hendries)	C						
INFANT FORMULA:							
Similac, powder	C		M				
INSTANT BREAKFAST:							
(Pillsbury):							
Chocolate	C		M		P	S	W
Chocolate Malt	C		M		P	S	W
Strawberry	C		M		P	S	W
Vanilla	C		M		P	S	W

Food Item	CORN	EGGS	MILK	NUTS	PEANUT	SOY	WHEAT

J

JAM/JELLY:
  (Knott's):

Concord Grape Jelly	C						
Mint Flavored Apple Jelly	C						
Orange Marmalade	C						
Red Raspberry Preserves	C						
Strawberry Preserves	C						

  (Polaner):

All Fruit, Apricot							
Fancy Fruit, Seedless Blackberry	C						
Sweet Orange Marmalade	C						

  (Raffetto) Jelly:

Burgundy Wine	C						
Condi-Mint	C						
Guava	C						
Icy Mint	C						
Mint	C						
Port Wine	C						
Sherry Wine	C						

  (Smucker's):

Apple Butter	C						
Apricot Preserves	C						
Concord Grape Jelly	C						
Orange Marmalade	C						
Strawberry Preserves	C						

  Sorrell Ridge:

Apple Cider							
Apricot							
Black Raspberry							
Blackberry							
Cherry Orange							
Concord Grape							
Cranberry							
Orange Marmalade							

Food Item	CORN	EGGS	MILK	NUTS	PEANUT	SOY	WHEAT
Peach							
Pear Apple							
Pineapple							
Raspberry							
Strawberry							
Wild Blueberry							
(Walnut Acres):							
Black Raspberry							
Blueberry Preserves							
Fruit Conserves:							
Apricot							
Orange Marmalade							
Raspberry							
Strawberry Jam							
Wild Blackberry							
Wild Elderberry							
JAM/JELLY, artificially sweetened:							
(Smucker's):							
Imitation Grape Jelly	C						
Imitation Strawberry Jam	C						
JUICE, asceptically packaged:							
(Minute Maid):							
Apple							
Grape							
Orange							
JUICE, bottled and canned (see also							
FRUIT JUICE):							
Apricot Nectar (Heart's Delight)	C						
Juicy Juice:							
Cherry							
Golden Good							
(Lakewood):							
Apple-Black Cherry							
Apple-Loganberry							
Black Cherry							
Cranberry Citrus Blend							
Mango							
Orange-Pineapple							
Passion Fruit							
Peaches 'n Creme							

Food Item	CORN	EGGS	MILK	NUTS	PEANUT	SOY	WHEAT
Piña Colada							
Pineapple							
Sparkling Grape							
Sparkling Loganberry							
Sparkling Orange							
Three Berry							
Snapple:							
Apple Crisp							
Apple 'n Cherry							
Apple 'n Cranberry							
Apple 'n Strawberry							
Orange							
Orange Supreme							
Papaya Holiday							
Raspberry Royale							
Straight Grape							
Vitamin Supreme	C						
V-8, no salt	C						
(Wagners) Papaya Concentrates:							
Creamed							
Hawaiian							
(Walnut Acres):							
Apple							
Cranberry Nectar:							
Unsweetened							
With Honey							
Purple Grape							
Super Veggie							
Vegetable Juice Cocktail							
JUICE, frozen concentrate:							
(Minute Maid):							
Apple							
Country Style Orange							
Grapefruit							
Orange							
Pineapple							
Pineapple-Orange							
Pink Grapefruit							
Reduced Acid Orange	C						
Tangerine							

Food Item	CORN	EGGS	MILK	NUTS	PEANUT	SOY	WHEAT
JUICY JUICE (See **JUICE**)							
JUNKET, RENNET CUSTARD:							
Chocolate	C		M				W
Dutch Chocolate	C		M		P	S	
Raspberry	C		M				
Strawberry	C		M				
Vanilla	C		M		P	S	
JUNKET, RENNET TABLETS	C		M		P	S	

Food Item	CORN	EGGS	MILK	NUTS	PEANUT	SOY	WHEAT

K

KARO SYRUP (See **SYRUP**)
KENTUCKY FRIED CHICKEN:

Food Item	CORN	EGGS	MILK	NUTS	PEANUT	SOY	WHEAT
Barbeque Sauce	C					S	W
Fat used for frying	C					S	
Hot Sauce	C		M			S	W
KETCHUP:							
(Del Monte)	C						W
(Health Valley Foods):							
Catch-Up:							
No-salt							
Regular							
(Heinz)	C						W
(Hunt's):							
No salt added	C						W
Regular	C						W
(Walnut Acres):							
Salted	C						W
Unsalted	C						W
KIELBASA/POLISH SAUSAGE:							
(Hillshire Farm):							
Polish Sausage	C					S	W
Polska Kielbasa:							
Beef	C					S	W
Mild	C					S	W
Regular	C					S	W
(Hormel):							
Kolbase Polish Sausage	C						
Polish Sausage	C		M			S	W
Skinless Kielbasa Polish Sausage	C		M			S	W
KIKKOMAN:							
Instant Soup:							
Aka Miso	C					S	W
Egg Flower Soup:							
Corn	C		M			S	W

Food Item	CORN	EGGS	MILK	NUTS	PEANUT	SOY	WHEAT
Hot & Sour	C		M			S	W
Shrimp	C					S	W
Vegetable	C		M			S	W
Osuimono	C					S	W
Shiro Miso	C					S	W
Tofu Miso	C					S	W
Wakame (seaweed)	C					S	W
Parchment:							
Chicken	C		M			S	W
Seafood	C				P	S	W
Seasoning Mixes:							
Chow Mein	C		M			S	W
Fried Rice	C		M			S	W
Meat Marinade	C		M			S	W
Salad Dressing:							
Creamy Oriental	C					S	W
Soy Sesame	C					S	W
Stir-Fry	C		M			S	W
Sweet & Sour	C					S	W
Teriyaki	C		M			S	W
Soy Sauce:							
Lite			M			S	W
Regular						S	W
Steak Sauce	C		M			S	W
Sukiyaki Sauce	C		M			S	W
Sweet & Sour Sauce	C					S	W
Tempura Sauce	C		M			S	W
Teriyaki Sauce:							
Baste & Glaze	C					S	W
Regular	C					S	W
KNISHES, POTATO:							
Frozen (Cohen's)	C	E			P	S	W
KNOCKWURST:							
(Health Valley Foods) Beef							
(Hillshire Farm)	C						
KOLLN (See **CEREALS**)							
KOOL-AID (See **DRINK MIX,**							
FRUIT DRINKS)							

Food Item	CORN	EGGS	MILK	NUTS	PEANUT	SOY	WHEAT

L

LACTAID:
Liquid | C | | | | P | S | |
Tablets
LECITHIN:
(Fearn):
  Liquid | | | | | | S | |
  Mint Flavored Liquid | | | | | | S | |
LE MENU, frozen dinners:
Chicken Cordon Bleu | C | E | M | N | P | S | W |
Ham Steak | C | | M | | P | S | W |
LEMON JUICE:
(Concord) *Squeez-eez:*
  Imitation | C | | | | | | |
  Reconstituted
LEMONADE (See FRUIT DRINKS, DRINK MIX)
LIME JUICE:
(Concord) *Squeez-eez:*
  Imitation | C | | | | | | |
  Reconstituted
(Giroux) Sweetened | C | | | | | | |
LIVERWURST/ BRAUNSCHWEIGER:
Braunschweiger (Hormel) | C | | M | | | | |
LOUIS RICH (See TURKEY, prepared)
LUNCHEON MEATS (See also individual meats):
Bologna (Hormel):
  Coarse Ground Beef Bologna | C | | M | | | S | W |
  Coarse Ground Bologna | C | | M | | | S | |
  Fine Ground Bologna | C | | M | | | S | |
  Braunschweiger (Hormel) | C | | M | | | | |
(Health Valley Foods):
  Beef:
    Bologna

Food Item	CORN	EGGS	MILK	NUTS	PEANUT	SOY	WHEAT
Salami							
Chicken:							
Bologna							
(Hormel) Perma-Fresh Lunch Meats:							
BBQ Loaf	C		M			S	
Beef Bologna	C						
Black Peppered Ham							
Bologna	C						W
Breast of Turkey	C		M			S	W
Buffet Loaf	C		M			S	W
Chopped Ham							
Cooked Ham	C		M				
Cotto Salami	C		M			S	
Genoa Salami	C		M				
Ham & Cheese Loaf	C		M			S	
Hard Salami			M				
Honey Loaf			M			S	W
(Iowa) Loaf			M			S	W
(Milwaukee) Smoky Thuringer		E	M			S	W
(New England) Luncheon Meat	C						
Olive Loaf	C		M			S	
Pickle Loaf	C		M			S	
Smoked Cooked Ham						S	W
Spiced Luncheon Meat	C		M			S	
(Oscar Mayer):							
Bar-B-Q Loaf	C		M				W
Beef Summer Sausage			M				
Bologna:							
Beef Bologna	C						
Beef Lebanon Bologna			M				
Bologna	C						
Bologna with Cheese	C		M				
Garlic Bologna, Beef	C						
Braunschweiger Liver Sausage	C						
Canadian Style Bacon							
Corned Beef							
Ham:							
Chopped Ham	C						
Cracked Black Pepper Ham							
Ham & Cheese Loaf	C		M				

Food Item	CORN	EGGS	MILK	NUTS	PEANUT	SOY	WHEAT
Honey Ham							
Italian Style Cooked Ham	C					S	
Smoked Cooked Ham							
Head Cheese	C						
Honey Loaf	C		M				
Italian Style Beef	C		M				
Liver Cheese	C						
Luncheon Meat	C						
Luxury Loaf	C		M				
New England Brand Sausage	C						
Old Fashioned Loaf	C		M			S	
Olive Loaf	C		M				
Peppered Loaf	C		M				
Pickle & Pimento Loaf	C		M				
Picnic Loaf	C		M				
Pastrami							W
Salami:							
Beef Cotto Salami	C						
Beef Salami for Beef	C					S	
Cotto Salami	C						
Genoa Salami			M				
Hard Salami			M				
Salami for Beer	C					S	
Smoked Chicken Breast	C					S	
Smoked Turkey Breast	C					S	
Summer Sausage			M				
Turkey:							
(Bil Mar):							
Breast of Turkey							
Mr. Turkey:							
Deli-pack Chubs:							
Barbecued Breast	C						
Smoked Breast	C					S	W
Other Lunch Meats:							
Bologna	C						
Chopped Ham	C					S	W
Cotto Salami	C					S	W
Pastrami	C						
Red Rind Bologna	C						
Smoked Ham	C					S	W

Food Item	C O R N	E G G S	M I L K	N U T S	P E A N U T	S O Y	W H E A T
Smoked Turkey	C						
Smoked Turkey Breast	C					S	W
Spiced Luncheon Loaf	C						
Turkey Breast							
Louis Rich:							
Oven Roasted Chicken Breast			M				
Oven Roasted Turkey Breast	C						
Smoked Turkey							
Smoked Turkey Breast							
Turkey Bologna							
Turkey Cotto Salami							
Turkey Ham							
Turkey Ham, chopped							
Turkey Luncheon Loaf							
Turkey Pastrami							
Turkey Salami							
Turkey Summer Sausage	C		M				

Food Item	CORN	EGGS	MILK	NUTS	PEANUT	SOY	WHEAT

M

McDONALD'S:

Breakfast Danish Pastry:

Food Item	CORN	EGGS	MILK	NUTS	PEANUT	SOY	WHEAT
Apple	C	E	M		P	S	W
Iced Cheese	C	E	M		P	S	W
Cinnamon Raisin	C	E	M		P	S	W
Raspberry	C	E	M		P	S	W

Breakfast Foods:

Food Item	CORN	EGGS	MILK	NUTS	PEANUT	SOY	WHEAT
Bacon							
Biscuit Dressing	C	E			P	S	
Butter			M				
Buttermilk Biscuits			M			S	W
Buttermilk Biscuits with Dressing	C	E	M		P	S	W
Canadian-style Bacon	C						
Cheese	C		M				
Egg McMuffin (muffin, egg, cheese, Canadian-style bacon)	C	E	M		P	S	W
English Muffin:	C		M		P	S	W
Grape Jam	C						
Strawberry Preserves	C						
Hash Browns	C				P	S	W
Hot Cakes:	C	E	M		P	S	W
Hot Cake Syrup	C		M				W
Whipped Butter Pats			M				
Pork Sausage	C					S	W

Birthday Cakes:

Food Item	CORN	EGGS	MILK	NUTS	PEANUT	SOY	WHEAT
Chocolate Cake	C	E	M		P	S	W
Yellow Cake	C	E	M		P	S	W
White Icing	C		M		P	S	

Condiments:

Food Item	CORN	EGGS	MILK	NUTS	PEANUT	SOY	WHEAT
Barbecue Sauce	C		M			S	W
Big Mac Sauce	C	E				S	W
Honey							
Hot Mustard Sauce	C	E	M			S	W
Ketchup	C						W

Food Item	CORN	EGGS	MILK	NUTS	PEANUT	SOY	WHEAT
Mayonnaise	C	E				S	W
Mustard	C						W
Onions, dehydrated							
Pickles	C						W
Sweet & Sour Sauce	C					S	W
Tartar Sauce	C	E				S	W
Cookies:							
Chocolaty Chip	C	E	M		P	S	W
McDonaldland	C	E			P	S	W
French Fries	C				P	S	
Hot Beverages:							
Coffee							
Hot Chocolate Drink	C	E	M		P	S	
Tea							
Hot Pie, Apple	C		M		P	S	W
Ice Cream & Sundaes:							
Cake Cones	C					S	W
Hot Caramel Topping	C		M				
Hot Fudge Topping	C		M				W
Peanut Topping					P		
Soft Serve Mix	C		M		P	S	
Strawberry Topping	C						
Juice:							
Grapefruit							
Orange							
Meat, Chicken, & Fish:							
Beef Patty							
Buns	C		M		P	S	W
Chicken McNuggets	C		M		P	S	W
Filet-o-Fish Sandwich	C		M		P	S	W
Milkshakes:							
Chocolate	C		M				W
Strawberry	C		M				
Vanilla	C		M				W
Soft Drinks:							
Coca-Cola, Classic	C		M				W
Orange Drink	C				P	S	
Sprite	C						

MACARONI (See **PASTA, NOODLES**)

Food Item	CORN	EGGS	MILK	NUTS	PEANUT	SOY	WHEAT
MACARONI & CHEESE:							
Frozen:							
(Myers)	C		M		P	S	W
Packaged Mix:							
(Golden Grain):							
Macaroni & Cheddar	C		M			S	W
(Prince):							
Macaroni & Cheese	C		M				W
Twists & Cheddar	C		M				W
MALTED MILK:							
(Carnation) Chocolate	C		M		P	S	W
(Horlicks):							
Powder:							
Chocolate	C	E	M		P	S	W
Natural			M				W
Tablets:							
Chocolate			M				W
Natural			M				W
MANISCHEWITZ:							
Borscht:							
Low-calorie	C						
With beets	C						
Crackers:							
Garlic Tams	C					S	W
Onion Tams	C					S	W
Tam Tams	C					S	W
Tam Tams, no-salt	C					S	W
Wheat Tams	C					S	W
Gefilte fish, unsalted		E					W
Matzo (See **MATZO**)							
Potato Starch							
Seltzer							
Soup Mixes:							
Minestrone	C					S	W
Split Pea	C					S	W
Vegetable		E					W
***MANWICH* SAUCE** (Hunt's)	C						W
MAPLE SYRUP (See **SYRUP**)							
MARINADE:							
Mr. Marinade:							

Food Item	CORN	EGGS	MILK	NUTS	PEANUT	SOY	WHEAT
Red Wine	C					S	W
Teriyaki with Wine	C		M			S	W
White Wine	C		M			S	W
(Premier Japan):							
Brown Rice Miso						S	
Miso Marinade	C					S	W
Mugi Miso						S	W
Shoyu Marinade	C					S	W
MATZO:							
(Goodman's):							
Whole Wheat							W
(Manischewitz):							
American	C					S	W
Daily Thin Tea							W
Dietetic, Thins							W
Egg 'n Onion	C	E					W
Matzo Farfel, daily							W
Matzo Meal							W
Matzo Miniatures, crackers:							
Matzo Cracker							W
Passover Egg		E					W
Wheat							W
Passover							W
Passover, Egg		E					W
Unsalted							W
Whole Wheat with Bran							W
MARGARINE:							
Blue Bonnet:							
Bakers Blend			M			S	
Butter Blend:							
Soft			M			S	
Stick			M			S	
Unsalted, stick			M			S	
Diet						S	
Regular, stick			M			S	
Soft			M			S	
Soft Whipped			M			S	
Spread:							
52% fat			M			S	
70% fat, stick			M			S	

Food Item	CORN	EGGS	MILK	NUTS	PEANUT	SOY	WHEAT
75% fat, stick			M			S	
Whipped, stick			M			S	
Fleischmann's:							
Diet	C					S	
Diet with Lite Salt	C					S	
Light Corn Oil Spread:							
Soft	C		M			S	
Stick	C		M			S	
Liquid Corn Oil	C		M			S	
Regular, stick	C		M			S	
Soft	C		M			S	
Squeeze	C		M			S	
Sweet, unsalted, Pareve	C					S	
Unsalted, stick	C					S	
Whipped	C		M			S	
Whipped, unsalted	C		M			S	
(Land O Lakes):							
Corn Oil	C		M		P	S	
Regular, sticks	C		M		P	S	
Soft	C		M		P	S	
Mazola, Corn Oil Margarine:							
Diet, Reduced Calorie	C					S	
Regular	C		M			S	
Unsalted	C					S	
(Weight Watchers):							
Soft	C	E			P	S	
Soft, unsalted	C	E			P	S	
Sticks	C				P	S	
MAYONNAISE:							
(Best Foods)		E				S	
(Health Valley Foods)	C	E				S	W
(Hellmann's)		E				S	
(Weight Watchers):							
Low Sodium	C	E				S	W
Regular	C	E				S	W
MAZOLA (See **OIL**)							
MEATBALL SEASONING MIX:							
(Tempo):							
Italian	C	E	M		P	S	W
Swedish	C	E	M		P	S	W

Food Item	CORN	EGGS	MILK	NUTS	PEANUT	SOY	WHEAT
MEAT FOOD, POTTED:							
(Hormel)			M			S	
MEAT LOAF SEASONING MIX:							
(Tempo)	C	E	M		P	S	W
MEAT SPREADS:							
(Oscar Mayer):							
Braunschweiger Liver Sausage	C						
Chili Con Carne Concentrate	C						W
German Brand Braunschweiger							
Ham & Cheese			M				
Ham Salad	C	E			P	S	
Sandwich Spread	C	E			P	S	
MERINGUE POWDER:							
(Wilton)	C	E	M				W
METHYLCELLULOSE:							
(Ener-G Foods)							
MILK, CHOCOLATE:							
Farm Best:							
Lowfat			M				
Whole			M				
Flav-O-Rich:							
1% milkfat	C		M				W
3.5% milkfat	C		M				W
3.25% milkfat	C		M				W
MILK, DRY:							
(Ener-G Foods):							
Cultured Buttermilk, powdered			M				
(Fearn) Non-Fat Dry Milk			M				
MILK, EVAPORATED, canned:							
(Carnation)							
MILLET (Ener-G Foods)							W
MIRIN:							
(Premier Japan), rice cooking wine	C						
MISO:							
(Erewhon):							
Genmai						S	
Hatcho						S	
Kome						S	
Mugi						S	W

Food Item	C O R N	E G G S	M I L K	N U T S	P E A N U T	S O Y	W H E A T
(Walnut Acres):							
Kome Miso						S	
MOUSSE MIX:							
Artificially Sweetened:							
San Sucre de Paris (Bernard):							
Cheesecake	C		M		P	S	W
Chocolate	C		M		P	S	W
Lemon	C		M		P	S	W
Strawberry	C		M		P	S	W
Regular:							
Rich & Luscious (Jell-O):							
Chocolate	C	E	M		P	S	
Chocolate Fudge	C	E	M		P	S	
MUFFIN MIX:							
Blueberry:							
(Duncan Hines) wild	C					S	W
(Walnut Acres)	C		M			S	W
Bran:							
& Honey (Duncan Hines)	C		M			S	W
(Fearn)			M			S	W
With Dates (Jiffy)						S	W
(Walnut Acres)	C		M				W
(Washington)	C		M			S	W
Corn:							
(Dromedary)	C					S	W
(Walnut Acres)	C		M			S	W
Maple Granola (Walnut Acres)	C		M	N	P	S	W
Pecan:							
(Duncan Hines)	C			N		S	W
Raisin:							
'n Spice (Duncan Hines)	C					S	W
MUFFINS:							
English:							
(Pepperidge Farm)	C	E	M		P	S	W
(Placentia)	C		M		P	S	W
(Thomas'):							
Honey Wheat	C				P	S	W
Raisin	C		M		P	S	W
Regular	C		M		P	S	W
Sourdough	C		M		P	S	W

Food Item	C O R N	E G G S	M I L K	N U T S	P E A N U T	S O Y	W H E A T
Frozen:							
(Pepperidge Farm)							
Cinnamon Swirl	C	E	M			S	W
Ready-to-Eat:							
(Ener-G Foods) Date Muffins							
(Entenmann's) *Fruit and Fibre*							
Muffins:							
Cinnamon Apple Raisin		E	M			S	W
MUSHROOMS:							
(Premier Japan) Shitake							
MUSTARD, Prepared:							
(French's):							
Bold 'n Spicy	C						W
Dijon	C						W
Yellow	C						W
(Health Valley Foods)	C						W
(Kosciusko) Spicy Brown	C						W

Food Item	C O R N	E G G S	M I L K	N U T S	P E A N U T	S O Y	W H E A T
N							
NABISCO (See **COOKIES, CRACKERS**)							
NACHO CHIPS (See **SNACKS**)							
NOODLES, DRY: (See also **PASTA**):							
(China Bowl), Chinese Noodles	C						W
(Goodman's), Egg, all varieties		E					W
(Mueller's) Egg Noodles		E					W
(Premier Japan):							
Soba							W
Udon							W
NOODLES, INSTANT:							
(Premier Japan) Ramen Noodles:							
Brown Rice						S	W
Buckwheat						S	W
Pearl Barley						S	W
Wakame						S	W
NOODLES, INSTANT MIX:							
Cup O' Noodles (Nissin), soup:							
Beef	C	E	M			S	W
Beef/Onion	C	E	M			S	W
Chicken	C	E	M			S	W
Chicken Mushroom	C	E	M			S	W
Crab	C		M		P	S	W
Garden Vegetable	C	E	M			S	W
Pork	C	E	M			S	W
Shrimp	C	E	M			S	W
Oodles of Noodles (Nissin), soup:							
Beef	C		M			S	W
Chicken	C					S	W
Chicken Mushroom	C		M			S	W
Garden Vegetable	C					S	W
Oriental	C		M			S	W
Pork	C		M			S	W
Shrimp	C		M			S	W
Ramen Pride:							
Beef	C		M			S	W

Food Item	C O R N	E G G S	M I L K	N U T S	P E A N U T	S O Y	W H E A T
Chicken	C					S	W
Top Ramen (Nissin), soup:							
Beef	C		M			S	W
Chicken	C					S	W
Chicken Mushroom	C		M			S	W
Garden Vegetable	C					S	W
Oriental	C		M			S	W
Pork	C		M			S	W
Savory Onion	C					S	W
Shrimp	C		M			S	W
NOODLES, MIX:							
Deluxe Noodles and Sauce (Lipton):							
Alfredo	C	E	M			S	W
Parmesan		E	M				W
Stroganoff	C	E	M			S	W
Noodles and Sauce (Lipton):							
Beef	C	E	M			S	W
Butter	C	E	M			S	W
Butter & Herb	C	E	M			S	W
Cheese	C	E	M			S	W
Chicken	C	E	M			S	W
Sour Cream & Chives	C	E	M			S	W.
NUT CRUNCH:							
(Charles) Cashew Crunch	C		M	N			
NUTRI-TREAT (Weight Watchers):							
Chocolate	C		M		P	S	
Eggnog	C		M				
Strawberry	C		M				
Vanilla Marshmallow	C		M				
NUTS (See also **PEANUTS**):							
(Fisher) Cashew Halves				N	P		
(Walnut Acres) Dry Roasted:							
Pistachios				N			
Spanish Peanuts					P		
Tamari Almonds				N		S	W
Tamari Cashews				N		S	W
Tamari Mixed Nuts				N		S	W
Walnuts:							
(Diamond) shelled, canned	C			N			

Food Item	CORN	EGGS	MILK	NUTS	PEANUT	SOY	WHEAT

O

OATMEAL (See **CEREAL**)
OIL, SALAD or COOKING:

Food Item	CORN	EGGS	MILK	NUTS	PEANUT	SOY	WHEAT
Corn (Mazola)	C						
Crisco	C				P	S	
(Health Valley Foods):							
Best Blend	C					S	
Corn	C						
Olive							
Peanut					P		
Safflower							
Sesame							
Soy						S	
Sunflower							
Olive:							
(Ferrara) Extra Virgin							
Puritan						S	
OLD EL PASO, grocery products:							
Beef Enchiladas	C					S	W
Beef Taco Filling	C		M			S	W
Chili with Beans	C		M			S	W
Enchilada Sauce:							
Hot	C						W
Mild	C						W
Garbanzos							
Jalapeño Bean Dip	C						W
Mexe-Beans							
Nachips	C					S	
Peeled Green Chilies	C						
Pickled Jalapeños	C				P	S	W
Pinto Beans							
Refried Beans							
Spanish Rice	C					S	W
Taco Dinner:							
Sauce	C						W

Food Item	CORN	EGGS	MILK	NUTS	PEANUT	SOY	WHEAT
Seasoning	C						
Shells	C					S	
Taco Dip	C						W
Taco Sauce:							
Hot	C						W
Mild	C						W
Taco Shells	C					S	
Tamales	C						W
Tamales with Chili Gravy	C						W
Tomatoes & Green Chilies							
Tomatoes & Jalapeños							
Tortillas, canned	C						
Tostada Shells	C					S	
OLIVE OIL (See **OIL**)							
OLIVES:							
Martini Olives (Raffetto)			M				
ONION RINGS, frozen:							
(Mrs. Paul's) Crispy	C		M			S	W
ONIONS, COCKTAIL:							
(Raffetto)	C						W
ONIONS, frozen:							
(Ore-Ida):							
Chopped Onions							
Onion Ringers	C					S	W
ORANGE JUICE:							
Dairy-Pak:							
Citrus Hill							
Tropicana							
(Minute Maid):							
Country Style							
From Concentrate							
Frozen Concentrate:							
(Minute Maid):							
Country Style							
Reduced Acid	C						
Regular							
OSCAR MAYER:							
Bacon:							
Bacon Bits							
Center Cut							

Food Item	CORN	EGGS	MILK	NUTS	PEANUT	SOY	WHEAT
Regular							
Thick Slice							
Breakfast Strips, *Lean 'N Tasty:*							
Beef						S	
Pork						S	
Frankfurters/Wieners:							
Beef Franks	C						
Hot Dogs:							
Bacon & Cheddar Cheese	C		M				
Cheese	C		M				
Nacho Cheese	C		M				
Little Wieners	C						
Wieners	C						
Ham:							
Boneless Jubilee							
Jubilee, canned							
Jubilee, slice							
Jubilee, steaks							
Link Sausage:							
Beef Smokies	C					S	
Cheese Smokies	C		M			S	
Little Friers Pork	C						
Little Smokies	C					S	
Smokie Links	C					S	
Meat Spreads:							
Braunschweiger Liver Sausage	C						
Chili Con Carne Concentrate	C						W
German Brand Braunschweiger							
Ham & Cheese			M				
Ham Salad	C	E			P	S	
Sandwich Spread	C	E			P	S	
Sliced Meats:							
Bar-B-Q Loaf	C		M				W
Beef Bologna	C						
Beef Cotto Salami	C						
Beef Lebanon Bologna			M				
Beef Salami for Beef	C					S	
Beef Summer Sausage			M				
Braunschweiger Liver Sausage	C						
Canadian Style Bacon							

Food Item	CORN	EGGS	MILK	NUTS	PEANUT	SOY	WHEAT
Chopped Ham	C						
Corned Beef							
Cotto Salami	C						
Cracked Black Pepper Ham							
Garlic Bologna, Beef	C						
Genoa Salami			M				
Ham & Cheese Loaf	C		M				
Hard Salami			M				
Head Cheese	C						
Honey Ham							
Honey Loaf	C		M				
Italian Style Cooked Ham	C					S	
Italian Style Beef	C		M				
Liver Cheese	C						
Luncheon Meat	C						
Luxury Loaf	C		M				
New England Brand Sausage	C						
Old Fashioned Loaf	C		M			S	
Olive Loaf	C		M				
Pastrami							W
Peppered Loaf	C		M				
Pickle and Pimento Loaf	C		M				
Picnic Loaf	C		M				
Salami for Beer	C					S	
Smoked Chicken Breast	C					S	
Smoked Cooked Ham							
Smoked Turkey Breast	C					S	
Summer Sausage			M				
OVALTINE	C		M		P	S	
OYSTER PIE, frozen (Myers)	C		M		P	S	W

Food Item	CORN	EGGS	MILK	NUTS	PEANUT	SOY	WHEAT

P

PANCAKE MIX, artificially sweetened:
(Sweet 'n Low):

Food Item	CORN	EGGS	MILK	NUTS	PEANUT	SOY	WHEAT
Pancake & Crepe	C	E	M		P	S	W
Potato Pancake	C	E				S	W

PANCAKE MIX, regular
(See also **BAKING MIX**):
(Arrowhead Mills):

Food Item	CORN	EGGS	MILK	NUTS	PEANUT	SOY	WHEAT
Buckwheat	C		M				W
Griddle Lite	C	E	M		P	S	
Multigrain	C		M				W
Triticale	C		M				W

Aunt Jemima:

Food Item	CORN	EGGS	MILK	NUTS	PEANUT	SOY	WHEAT
Buttermilk	C		M				W
Whole Wheat	C					S	W

(Fearn):

Food Item	CORN	EGGS	MILK	NUTS	PEANUT	SOY	WHEAT
Buckwheat						S	W
Rich Earth						S	W
7 Grain Buttermilk:							
Low-sodium	C		M			S	W
Regular	C		M			S	W
Soy-O						S	W
Whole wheat						S	W

(Health Valley Foods):

Food Item	CORN	EGGS	MILK	NUTS	PEANUT	SOY	WHEAT
Original Recipe							W
With Buttermilk			M				W

(Pepperidge Farm):

Food Item	CORN	EGGS	MILK	NUTS	PEANUT	SOY	WHEAT
Corn Pancake Mix	C		M				W

(Walnut Acres):

Food Item	CORN	EGGS	MILK	NUTS	PEANUT	SOY	WHEAT
Buckwheat	C		M				W
Buttermilk Johnny Cake	C		M			S	
Hi-Bran	C		M			S	W
Rice	C					S	
12 Grain	C		M			S	W
Unbleached White with Soy	C		M			S	W
Wheatless	C		M			S	W

Food Item	CORN	EGGS	MILK	NUTS	PEANUT	SOY	WHEAT
Whole Wheat with Soy	C		M			S	W
PARCHMENT:							
(Kikkoman):							
Chicken	C		M			S	W
Seafood	C				P	S	W
PASTA (See also **NOODLES**):							
(Butoni) Spinach Linguine							W
(DeBoies) Corn Pasta:							
Elbows	C						
Ribbons	C						
Shells	C						
Thin Spaghetti	C						
Ziti	C						
(Ener-G Foods):							
Aglutella Gluten-free, Wheat-free,							
Low Protein:							
Spaghetti	C				P	S	
Spaghetti Rings	C				P	S	
Macaroni	C				P	S	
Tagliatelle	C				P	S	
Aproten Gluten-free, Wheat-free,							
Low Protein:							
Anellini	C				P	S	
Ditalini	C				P	S	
Rigatini	C				P	S	
Tagliatelle	C				P	S	
(Erewhon):							
40% Buckwheat Soba							W
80% Buckwheat Soba							W
Ramen Dashi						S	W
Ramen Pasta							W
Udon							W
(Health Valley Foods):							
Amaranth, spaghetti							W
Regular:							
Elbows	C						W
Lasagna	C						W
Spaghetti	C						W
With 4 Vegetables, elbows	C						W
With Spinach:							
Lasagna	C						W

Food Item	CORN	EGGS	MILK	NUTS	PEANUT	SOY	WHEAT
Spaghetti	C						W
(Mueller's):							
Spaghetti, Macaroni							W
Twist Trio							W
(Prince) enriched							W
Rotini Primavera							W
(Ronzoni) enriched							W
(Walnut Acres):							
Corn:							
Elbows	C						
Spaghetti	C						
Vegetable Elbow Macaroni							W
Whole Wheat:							
Egg Noodles		E					W
Elbow Macaroni							W
Sesame Spirals							W
Spaghetti							W
PASTA, canned:							
(Hormel):							
Lasagna	C		M			S	W
Macaroni & Cheese	C		M			S	W
Noodles & Beef	C		M			S	W
Noodles & Chicken, *Dinty Moore*	C		M			S	W
Spaghetti & Beef	C		M			S	W
Spaghetti & Meatballs	C		M			S	W
(Walnut Acres):							
Noodles & Ground Beef			M			S	W
PASTA MIX (See also **NOODLES**):							
Pasta and Sauce (Lipton):							
Creamy Garlic	C		M			S	W
Herb Tomato	C		M			S	W
PASTA ENTRÉES, frozen:							
(Health Valley Foods):							
Lean Living Dinners:							
Spinach Lasagna			M				W
Meals For Two:							
Spinach Lasagna			M			S	W
(Ronzoni):							
Cheese Manicotti	C		M			S	W
(Stouffer's):							
Fettucini Primavera	C	E	M		P		W

Food Item	CORN	EGGS	MILK	NUTS	PEANUT	SOY	WHEAT
Lean Cuisine:							
Cheese Cannelloni	C	E	M		P		W
Linguine with Pesto Sauce	C		M	N	P		W
Noodles Romanoff	C	E	M		P		W
Macaroni & Cheese	C	E	M		P		W
PASTA MEALS (Ragu):							
Shells in Sauce, with Beef	C		M				W
Spaghetti in Sauce	C		M				W
Twists in Sauce	C		M				W
PASTA SAUCES (See also							
SPAGHETTI SAUCE):							
(Walnut Acres):							
Clam							W
Marinara			M			S	W
Spaghetti			M				W
PEACHES (See **FRUIT, CANNED**)							
PEANUT BRITTLE:							
(Charles)	C				P		
PEANUT BUTTER:							
(Arrowhead Mills):							
Creamy					P		
Crunchy					P		
(Erewhon) salted and unsalted:							
Chunky					P		
Creamy					P		
(Health Valley Foods):							
All varieties					P		
Jif:							
Creamy	C				P	S	
Crunchy	C				P	S	
Peter Pan:							
Creamy	C				P	S	
Skippy:							
Creamy	C				P		
Super Chunk	C				P		
(Walnut Acres):							
Chunk Roasted					P		
Roasted					P		
PEANUT BUTTER CHIPS:							
(Reese's)	C		M		P	S	

Food Item	CORN	EGGS	MILK	NUTS	PEANUT	SOY	WHEAT
PEANUT BUTTER SPREADS:							
(Walnut Acres):							
Banana Peanut					P		
Date Peanut					P		
Peanut Butter Honey					P		
Peanut Butter, Honey, Sesame					P		
PEANUTS:							
Butter Toasted (Charles)			M		P		
Caramel-coated:							
(Planters) *Sweet 'n Crunchy*			M		P		
(Fisher):							
Party Peanuts					P		
Honey Roasted:							
(Eagle) *Honey Roast*	C				P		W
(Planters)	C				P		
PEAS, canned:							
(Del Monte)							
PEAS, frozen:							
(Birds Eye) Sugar Snap							
PECTIN:							
Jell-Set (Concord)	C						
Slim Set (Iroquois)	C						W
(Walnut Acres) Low Methoxyl							
PEPPERIDGE FARM:							
Layer Cake:							
Chocolate Fudge	C	E	M		P	S	W
Golden	C	E	M		P	S	W
PEPPERONI:							
(Hormel):							
Chunk Pepperoni			M				
Pepperoni		E	M				
Rosa Pepperoni			M				W
Rosa Grande Pepperoni			M			S	W
Sliced Pepperoni			M				
PEPPERS:							
Hot:							
(Victoria) Stuffed Cherry	C	E	M		P	S	W
(Old El Paso):							
Peeled Green Chilies	C						
Pickled Jalapeños	C				P	S	W

Food Item	CORN	EGGS	MILK	NUTS	PEANUT	SOY	WHEAT
PESTO, frozen:							
Pesto For Pasta (Armanino Farms)	C		M		P	S	
PICKLE RELISH (See **PICKLES**)							
PICKLES/PICKLED FRUITS							
& VEGETABLES:							
(B an' G) Kosher Dill Gerkins,							
No salt	C						W
(Heinz):							
Sweet Relish	C						W
(Premier Japan):							
Takuan (radish pickles)							
(Raffetto):							
Baby Corn Cobs	C						W
Gherkins	C						W
Mustard *Medley*	C						W
Pickled *Medley*	C			N			W
Pickled Watermelon:							
Plantation Circles	C						W
Plantation Cubes							
Plantation Cubes & Cantaloupe	C						W
Relish:							
Corn Relish	C						W
Harlequin Relish	C						W
Onion Relish	C						W
Pepper Relish	C						W
Watermelon Relish	C						W
Refrigerated (Claussen):							
Bread 'n Butter	C						W
Kosher Dills	C						W
No-garlic Dills	C						W
Pickle Relish	C						W
Sauerkraut							
Sweet Pickles	C						W
Tomatoes	C						W
PIE:							
(Entenmann's):							
Blueberry Crumb Pie	C		M	N		S	W
Lemon Pie	C	E	M			S	W
PIE CRUST, CHOCOLATE:							
(Keebler) *Ready-Crust*	C	E	M		P	S	W

Food Item	CORN	EGGS	MILK	NUTS	PEANUT	SOY	WHEAT
PIE CRUST, frozen:							
(Mrs. Smith's) deep dish			M			S	W
(Pet) deep dish	C		M			S	W
PIE CRUST, GRAHAM CRACKER:							
(Keebler) *Ready-Crust*	C	E			P	S	W
PIE FILLING (See also **PUDDING & PIE FILLING**):							
Canned:							
(Comstock) Cherry	C						W
PIE GLAZE & FILLING MIX:							
(Salada):							
Danish-style:							
Raspberry	C				P	S	
Strawberry	C				P	S	
Easy As Pie:							
Blueberry	C						
Peach	C						
Strawberry	C						
PIE GLAZE MIX:							
Glaze a Pie! (Concord):							
Blueberry	C						W
Peach	C						W
Strawberry	C						W
Reddy Glaze (Concord):							
Strawberry	C						W
PIE MIX:							
(Jell-O):							
Chocolate Mousse	C	E	M		P	S	W
Royal *No-Bake:*							
Chocolate Mousse	C	E	M		P	S	W
Lemon Meringue	C	E	M			S	W
PIEROGIES, frozen:							
(Golden) Potato & Cheese	C		M		P	S	W
(Mrs. T's):							
Potato & Cheese	C	E	M		P	S	W
Potato & Onion	C	E	M		P	S	W
PIGS' FEET, PICKLED:							
(Hormel)		E	M			S	W
PIGS' KNUCKLES, PICKLED:							
(Victoria) Boneless	C						W

Food Item	C O R N	E G G S	M I L K	N U T S	P E A N U T	S O Y	W H E A T
PIMIENTOS:							
(Dromedary)							
PINEAPPLE (See **FRUIT**)							
PIZZA, FROZEN:							
(Buitoni):							
Instant	C	E	M			S	W
Slices	C		M		P	S	W
(Ellio's):							
French Bread	C	E	M		P	S	W
Slices	C		M			S	W
(Stouffer's) French Bread	C		M		P	S	W
PIZZA BITES (Matlaw's), cheese	C	E	M			S	W
PIZZA ROLLS (Jeno's), cheese	C	E	M			S	W
PIZZA SAUCE (Progresso)							
PIZZA SHELLS:							
Rice Pizza Shells (Ener-G Foods)	C					S	
POCKET FRUIT (Sunfield):							
Apricot	C						
POLISH SAUSAGE (See **KIELBASA**)							
POPCORN, ready-to-eat:							
Butter-flavored:							
(Utz's)	C						
Caramel Corn:							
(Bachman)	C	E	M		P	S	
(Charles)	C	E	M		P	S	
Caramel Crunch,							
(Orville Redenbacher's)	C	E	M		P	S	
Cheese:							
(Bachman)	C		M			S	W
(Charles)	C		M			S	W
(Utz's)	C		M			S	W
No-Salt:							
(Charles)	C					S	
Regular:							
(Bachman)	C					S	
(Charles)	C				P	S	
POPCORN, uncooked:							
(Cracker Jack)	C						
Jiffy Pop, natural flavor	C					S	

Food Item	CORN	EGGS	MILK	NUTS	PEANUT	SOY	WHEAT
POPEYES:							
Bar-b-que Sauce	C		M			S	W
Cajun Mustard Sauce	C					S	W
Sweet & Sour Sauce	C					S	W
POP-ICE (See **FROZEN DESSERTS & CONFECTIONS**)							
POP TARTS (See **TOASTER CAKE/ PASTRY**)							
POSTUM (General Foods)	C						W
POTATO CHIPS:							
(Bachman):							
BBQ	C		M		P	S	W
Hot Flavor	C				P	S	W
Regular	C				P	S	
Sour Cream & Onion	C		M		P	S	W
Unsalted	C				P	S	
Vinegar	C		M		P	S	
(Charles):							
Bacon 'N Cheddar	C		M			S	W
Bar-B-Q	C		M			S	W
No-Salt							
Regular							
Sour Cream, Onion, Chives	C		M			S	W
Waffle							
Delta Gold, dip style	C				P	S	
(Eagle Snacks):							
Crispy Cuts					P	S	
Lattice Sliced					P	S	
(Health Valley Foods):							
Country Chips							
Country Ripples							
No Salt, all varieties							
Regular							
O'Gradys	C				P	S	
(Pringles):							
Cheez-ums	C		M		P	S	W
Light	C				P	S	
Regular	C				P	S	
Rippled	C				P		
Sour Cream 'N Onion	C		M		P	S	W

Food Item	C O R N	E G G S	M I L K	N U T S	P E A N U T	S O Y	W H E A T
Ruffles:							
Cheddar & Jalapeño	C		M		P	S	W
Regular	C				P	S	
(Utz's):							
BBQ	C					S	W
Chesapeake Bay Seasoning	C					S	W
Grandma Utz Hand Cooked							
Home Style						S	
No Salt							
Red Hot	C					S	W
Regular							
Salt & Vinegar	C		M				
Sour Cream & Onion	C		M		P	S	W
(Wise):							
Regular	C					S	
Ridgies	C					S	
POTATO FLOUR:							
(Ener-G Foods):							
Fine Potato Flour							
POTATO ROLLS (Martin's)	C		M		P	S	W
POTATO STARCH:							
(Ener-G Foods)							
(Manischewitz)							
POTATO STICKS (Durkee)	C					S	
POTATO TOPPING Mix (Concord)	C				P	S	W
POTATOES, canned:							
(Hormel):							
Au Gratin Potatoes & Bacon	C		M			S	W
Dinty Moore:							
Hashed Potatoes & Beef						S	W
Scalloped Potatoes & Ham	C		M			S	W
POTATOES, frozen:							
(Ore-Ida):							
Cheddar Browns			M				
Cottage Fries						S	
Country Style Dinner Fries						S	
Crispers						S	
Crispy Crowns:							
Onion	C					S	W
Regular	C					S	W

Food Item	CORN	EGGS	MILK	NUTS	PEANUT	SOY	WHEAT
Golden Crinkles						S	
Golden Fries						S	
Golden Patties						S	
Heinz Deep Fries:							
Crinkle Cuts						S	
Regular Cuts						S	
Shoestrings						S	
Heinz Hash Browns with Butter							
Sauce & Onions			M			S	
Home Style Potato Wedges						S	
Lites:							
Crinkle Cuts						S	
Shoestrings						S	
Microwave:							
Crinkle Cuts						S	
Tater Tots						S	W
O'Brien Potatoes							
Pixie Crinkles						S	
Shoestrings						S	
Shredded Hash Browns							
Southern Style Hash Browns							
Tater Tots:							
Bacon						S	W
Onion						S	W
Regular						S	W
Whole Peeled Potatoes							
(Stouffer's):							
Scalloped Potatoes	C		M		P		W
POTATOES, instant:							
(Betty Crocker) *Potato Buds*	C				P	S	
(French's) Idaho Mashed	C				P	S	
POUND CAKE (See **CAKE**)							
PREMIER JAPAN:							
Brown Rice Crackers:							
Seaweed						S	
Sesame						S	
Brown Rice Malt Syrup							W
Brown Rice Vinegar							
Goma Furikake Black							
Goma Shio White (sesame seeds)							

Food Item	CORN	EGGS	MILK	NUTS	PEANUT	SOY	WHEAT
Kuzu (wild arrowroot starch)							
Marinades:							
Brown Rice Miso						S	
Miso Marinade	C					S	W
Mugi Miso						S	W
Shoyu Marinade	C					S	W
Mirin (rice cooking wine)	C						
Noodles:							
Soba							W
Udon							W
Pickled Ginger							
Quick Brown Rice Porridge							W
Quick Brown Rice with Vegetables							W
Ramen Noodles:							
Brown Rice						S	W
Buckwheat						S	W
Pearl Barley						S	W
Wakame						S	W
Roasted Black Sesame Seeds							
Seaweeds & Sea Vegetable Products:							
Agar-Agar Flakes							
Chopped Kombu							
Hijiki							
Instant Wakame							
Toasted Sushi Nori							
Soy Sauce:							
Mild Shoyu						S	W
Ponzu	C					S	W
Shoyu						S	W
Takuan (radish pickles)							
Tea Bags:							
Bancha							
Genmaicha							
Kukicha							
Toasted Sesame Oil							
Vegetables & Fruits:							
Azuki (beans)							
Shitake (mushrooms)							
Umeboshi (plums)							
Wasabi Powder (horseradish)							

Food Item	CORN	EGGS	MILK	NUTS	PEANUT	SOY	WHEAT
PRETZELS:							
(Anderson) all varieties	C					S	W
(Bachman):							
Butter Twist			M			S	W
Cheese Sticks	C		M			S	W
Hard							W
Petite						S	W
Regular						S	W
(Charles)							
Butter Thin	C		M			S	W
Cheese Pretzel Gems	C		M			S	W
Choco-Covered	C	E	M		P	S	W
Peanut Butter Pretzels	C		M		P	S	W
Pretzel Gems	C					S	W
Pretzel Logs	C					S	W
Pretzel Perfects	C	E	M		P	S	W
Pretzel Rods	C					S	W
Thick Pretzels	C					S	W
Thick Pretzels, no salt	C					S	W
Goldfish (Pepperidge Farm)						S	W
(Health Valley Foods):							
Natural	C						W
Whole Wheat	C						W
Mister Salty (Nabisco):							
Butter-flavored:							
Rings			M			S	W
Sticks			M			S	W
Twists			M			S	W
Dutch							W
Logs						S	W
Mini	C					S	W
Mini Mix	C					S	W
Nuggets						S	W
Pretzel Sticks						S	W
Rings						S	W
Rods						S	W
Twists						S	W
Veri-Thin Pretzel Sticks						S	W
(Reisman) Rods	C					S	W
Rold Gold, Twists	C					S	W

Food Item	C O R N	E G G S	M I L K	N U T S	P E A N U T	S O Y	W H E A T
(Utz's):							
Hard, Old-Fashioned							W
Thin, Wheel	C					S	W
PRETZELS, soft:							
Frozen:							
(Original Philadelphia)							W
Superpretzel (J & J)	C						W
PROSCIUTTO HAM:							
(Hormel)			M			S	W
PUDDING & PIE FILLING (See also							
JUNKET, CUSTARD MIX, MOUSSE MIX):							
Mix, instant:							
(Jell-O):							
Pistachio	C		M	N	P	S	
(Royal), regular:							
Banana Cream	C						
Butterscotch	C		M				
Chocolate	C						
Chocolate Mint	C						
Dark 'n Sweet	C						
Lemon	C						
Vanilla	C						
(Royal), sugar-free:							
Butterscotch	C		M				
Chocolate	C						
Vanilla	C		M				
Mix, to be cooked, regular							
(Jell-O):							
Americana:							
Golden Egg Custard	C	E	M				
Rice	C				P	S	
Vanilla Tapioca	C						
Chocolate	C						
(My-T-Fine):							
Chocolate	C					S	
Chocolate Fudge	C					S	
Vanilla	C					S	
(Royal):							
Banana Cream	C					S	
Butterscotch	C		M			S	

Food Item	CORN	EGGS	MILK	NUTS	PEANUT	SOY	WHEAT
Chocolate	C						
Dark 'n Sweet	C						
Flan with Caramel Sauce	C						
Key Lime	C					S	
Lemon	C					S	
Vanilla	C					S	
Vanilla Tapioca	C					S	
Refrigerated:							
(Axelrod's) Rice Pudding		E	M				
(Rich's):							
Butterscotch	C		M		P	S	W
Chocolate	C		M		P	S	W
Vanilla	C		M		P	S	W
PUDDING POPS (Jell-O), frozen:							
Chocolate-Vanilla Swirl	C		M		P	S	W
Vanilla	C		M		P	S	W
PUFF PASTRY:							
Frozen:							
(Pepperidge Farm)						S	W
PUMPKIN, canned:							
(Libby's)							

Food Item	C O R N	E G G S	M I L K	N U T S	P E A N U T	S O Y	W H E A T

Q

QUAKER MAID:
  Frozen Meat Products:

Food Item	C O R N	E G G S	M I L K	N U T S	P E A N U T	S O Y	W H E A T
Beef Patties							
Breaded Beef & Veal Patties						S	
Italian Meatballs	C		M			S	W
Sandwich Slices						S	
Sandwich Steaks							

QUIK (Nestlé):
  Powdered:

Food Item	C O R N	E G G S	M I L K	N U T S	P E A N U T	S O Y	W H E A T
Chocolate	C	E			P	S	
Strawberry	C						W
Sugar Free	C	E	M		P	S	
Syrup, Chocolate	C						

Food Item	C O R N	E G G S	M I L K	N U T S	P E A N U T	S O Y	W H E A T

R

RAMEN PRIDE (see **NOODLES**)
RELISH (See **PICKLES**)
RICE:
  Brown, long grain:
    (Mahatma)
    (River)
    (Uncle Ben's)
  White:
    Converted (Uncle Ben's)
    Enriched, long-grain:
      (Carolina) regular, instant
      (Mahatma) regular, instant
      (Success) precooked
    Enriched, medium-grain:
      (River)
      (Water Maid)

Food Item	CORN	EGGS	MILK	NUTS	PEANUT	SOY	WHEAT
RICE, canned:							
(Old El Paso):							
Spanish Rice	C					S	W
RICE SEASONING MIX:							
(Fantastic Foods) *Quick Pilaf:*							
Brown Rice with Miso						S	W
Spanish Brown Rice						S	W
Three Grain with Herbs	C					S	W
(Mahatma) Yellow Rice Mix	C					S	W
(Near East) Chicken Flavored	C						W
(Riviana) *Make-it-Easy:*							
Beef & Vermicelli	C		M			S	W
Chicken & Vermicelli	C					S	W
(Uncle Ben's):							
Brown & Wild Rice	C		M			S	W
Country Inn:							
Broccoli Au Gratin	C		M			S	W
Garden Style	C		M		P	S	W

Food Item	CORN	EGGS	MILK	NUTS	PEANUT	SOY	WHEAT
New England Style	C		M			S	W
Oriental with Vegetables	C		M			S	W
Royale, Chicken	C		M			S	W
Spanish Style with Cheese	C		M			S	
Long Grain & Wild Rice:							
Fast-Cooking	C		M			S	W
Original	C					S	W
(Walnut Acres):							
Bombay Rice					P		
Herbed Bulgur Rice				N			W
Oriental Rice						S	
Rice Pilaf						S	
Spanish Rice							
Three-Grain Rice Blend							
RICE & SAUCE (Lipton):							
Beef	C		M			S	W
Chicken	C					S	W
Herb & Butter	C		M			S	W
Mushroom	C		M			S	W
Rice Almondine	C		M	N		S	W
Rice Provencale	C		M			S	W
RICE-A-RONI:							
Chicken	C					S	W
Chicken & Mushroom	C		M			S	W
Herb & Butter	C		M			S	W
Pilaf	C					S	W
Spanish	C					S	W
RICE BRAN:							
(Ener-G Foods)							
RICE CAKES:							
(Chico-San):							
Plain							
With Buckwheat							W
With Corn	C						
With Millet							W
With Rye							W
With Sesame							
(Quaker):							
Sesame							
With Corn	C						

Food Item	CORN	EGGS	MILK	NUTS	PEANUT	SOY	WHEAT
RICE FLOUR:							
(Ener-G Foods):							
Brown Rice Flour							
Sweet Rice Flour							
White Rice Flour							
(Fearn)							
RICE POLISH:							
(Ener-G Foods)							
RICE PRODUCTS:							
(Amsnack):							
Brown Rice Thin Crackers			M				
Rice Chips:							
Almond				N			
Nacho Cheese			M				
Onion							
Plain							
Unsalted							
Rice Flakes			M				
(Premier Japan):							
Brown Rice Malt Syrup							W
Brown Rice Vinegar							
Quick Brown Rice Porridge							W
Quick Brown Rice with Vegetable							W
RICE STARCH:							
(Ener-G Foods)							
RICE SYRUP:							
Yinnies (Chico San)	C						W
ROAST BEEF HASH:							
Mary Kitchen						S	W
ROLL/BUN DOUGH:							
Refrigerated:							
(Pillsbury):							
Cinnamon	C		M		P	S	W
Crescent	C				P	S	W
Orange Danish	C		M		P	S	W
(Sun-Maid) Raisin Cinnamon	C	E	M		P	S	W
ROLLS/BUNS:							
(Pepperidge Farm):							
Butter Crescent			M				W
Club	C				P	S	W

Food Item	CORN	EGGS	MILK	NUTS	PEANUT	SOY	WHEAT
Croissant Sandwich	C	E	M		P	S	W
Hamburger	C	E	M		P	S	W
Sourdough French	C				P	S	W
ROLLS, SWEET:							
(Aunt Fanny's) *Pecan Twirls*	C	E		N	P	S	W
RONZONI (See **PASTA**)							
ROY ROGERS:							
Roast Beef	C					S	W
Sauces:							
BBQ	C		M			S	W
Horseradish	C	E				S	W
Sweet 'n Sour	C		M				W

Food Item	CORN	EGGS	MILK	NUTS	PEANUT	SOY	WHEAT

S

SALAD DRESSING, regular:
  Bottled, reduced calorie:
    Magic Mountain, no oil:

Food Item	CORN	EGGS	MILK	NUTS	PEANUT	SOY	WHEAT
Bleu Cheese	C		M				W
Cucumber Yogurt	C						W
French-Style	C		M		P	S	W
Herb & Spice	C						W
Northern Italian	C						W
Onion & Chive	C						W

    Marie's:

Food Item	CORN	EGGS	MILK	NUTS	PEANUT	SOY	WHEAT
Reduced Calorie, Blue Cheese	C	E	M			S	W

    Pfeiffer:

Food Item	CORN	EGGS	MILK	NUTS	PEANUT	SOY	WHEAT
Caesar	C		M			S	W
Red Wine Vinegar & Oil	C					S	W

    (Walden Farms), reduced calorie:

Food Item	CORN	EGGS	MILK	NUTS	PEANUT	SOY	WHEAT
Bleu Cheese	C	E	M			S	W
French	C	E				S	W
Italian:							
Low Sodium	C					S	W
No Sugar Added	C					S	W
Regular	C					S	W
Thousand Island	C	E				S	W

    (Weight Watchers):

Food Item	CORN	EGGS	MILK	NUTS	PEANUT	SOY	WHEAT
Thousand Island Dressing	C	E				S	W

    (Wish-Bone) *Lite:*

Food Item	CORN	EGGS	MILK	NUTS	PEANUT	SOY	WHEAT
Chunky Blue Cheese	C		M		P	S	W
French	C					S	W
Garden Medley	C					S	W
Italian	C					S	W

  Bottled, regular:
    (Health Valley Foods):

Food Item	CORN	EGGS	MILK	NUTS	PEANUT	SOY	WHEAT
Avocado	C	E	M		P	S	
Blue Cheese	C	E	M		P	S	
Creamy Yogurt	C	E	M		P	S	
Green Goddess	C	E	M		P	S	

Food Item	CORN	EGGS	MILK	NUTS	PEANUT	SOY	WHEAT
No-Salt:							
Avocado	C	E	M		P	S	
Original Herb	C	E	M		P	S	
1000 Island	C	E	M		P	S	
Original Herb	C	E	M		P	S	
Real Cheese & Herbs			M			S	
Real French						S	
Real Italian						S	
Roqeufort	C	E	M		P	S	
1000 Island	C	E	M		P	S	
(Knott's Berry Farm):							
Bleu Cheese	C	E	M			S	W
Creamy French	C	E				S	W
Creamy Italian	C					S	W
Creamy Ranch	C	E	M			S	W
Thousand Island	C	E				S	W
Marie's:							
Avocado Goddess	C	E	M			S	W
Blue Cheese	C	E	M			S	W
Buttermilk Spice	C	E	M			S	W
Creamy Bacon & Chive	C	E	M			S	W
Italian Garlic	C	E	M			S	W
Italian Herb & Romano	C	E	M			S	W
Italian with Cheese	C	E	M			S	W
Ranch	C	E	M			S	W
Russian	C	E	M			S	W
Thousand Island	C	E	M			S	W
Pfeiffer:							
Russian	C	E				S	W
Seven Seas:							
Creamy Russian	C					S	W
Green Goddess	C		M		P	S	W
Red Wine Vinegar & Oil	C					S	W
(Walnut Acres):							
Creamy Chive	C	E					W
Creamy French	C	E	E				W
Creamy Italian	C	E	E				W
Creamy Watercress	C	E					W
Italian	C						W
Spicy Spanish	C						W
Thousand Island	C	E					W

Food Item	C O R N	E G G S	M I L K	N U T S	P E A N U T	S O Y	W H E A T
(Wish-Bone):							
Chunky Blue Cheese	C		M		P	S	W
Creamy Italian	C		M			S	W
Creamy Romano & Parmesan	C	E	M			S	W
Deluxe French	C					S	W
Dijon Vinaigrette	C					S	W
Garlic French	C					S	W
Italian	C		M			S	W
Robusto Italian	C		M			S	W
Thousand Island	C	E				S	W
Vinaigrette	C					S	
SALAD DRESSING MIX:							
(Good Seasons) Lite Italian	C					S	W
(Kikkoman):							
Creamy Oriental	C					S	W
Soy Sesame	C					S	W
SALAMI (See LUNCHEON MEATS)							
SALT:							
(Morton) Iodized	C						
SALT SUBSTITUTE:							
Nu-Salt (Cumberland)							
SANDWICH SPRED (Hellmann's)	C	E				S	W
SARDINES:							
(King Oscar) in olive oil							
SAUCE MIX:							
(French's):							
Cheese	C		M			S	
Sour Cream	C		M				
Spaghetti, Italian-style	C		M				
Stroganoff	C		M			S	W
Sweet 'N Sour	C					S	W
Teriyaki	C					S	W
Hollandaise:							
(Concord)	C	E	M		P	S	W
(Knorr Swiss)	C		M		P	S	W
SAUCE, prepared:							
A.1. Steak Sauce	C		M				W
Alfredo Sauce (Ferrara)	C	E	M		P	S	W
Barbecue:							
(Enrico's) Mesquite Flavor						S	

Food Item	CORN	EGGS	MILK	NUTS	PEANUT	SOY	WHEAT
(Hunt's) *Thick & Rich:*							
New Orleans Style	C			N			W
Original Recipe	C						W
(Iroquois) *Texas Best*							
Regular	C		M			S	W
Thick 'n Rich	C		M			S	W
(Walnut Acres)	C						W
Cayenne Pepper:							
(Durkee) Frank's *Red Hot*	C						W
Cocktail:							
(Enrico's)							
Enchilada:							
(Old El Paso):							
Hot	C						W
Mild	C						W
(Raffetto):							
Brandi-Chef Sauce							
Duck Sauce	C						W
Ham Glaze	C						W
Mint Sauce	C		M				W
Salsa:							
(Enrico's) Salsa Picante:							
Hot							
Mild							
Hot Cha Cha, mild							
(Old El Paso) *Thick 'n Chunky*	C						W
Soy:							
(Arrowhead Mills) Tamari Soy						S	W
(Kikkoman):							
Lite			M			S	W
Regular						S	W
(La Choy)	C		M			S	W
(Premier Japan):							
Mild Shoyu						S	W
Ponzu	C					S	W
Shoyu						S	W
(Walnut Acres):							
Tamari Soy Sauce						S	W
Steak:							
(Kikkoman)	C		M			S	W

Food Item	CORN	EGGS	MILK	NUTS	PEANUT	SOY	WHEAT
(Lea & Perrins)	C						W
Sukiyaki Sauce:							
(Kikkoman)	C		M			S	W
Sweet & Sour:							
(Kikkoman)	C					S	W
(Polynesian) Spare Rib	C						W
Taco:							
(Old El Paso):							
Hot	C						W
Mild	C						W W
(Ortega), hot	C					S	W
Tartar (Hellmann's)		E				S	
Tempura Sauce:							
(Kikkoman)	C		M			S	W
Tobasco (McIlhenny)	C						W
Teriyaki:							
(Kikkoman):							
Baste & Glaze	C					S	W
Regular	C					S	W W
Worcestershire (Lea & Perrins)	C						W
SAUSAGE:							
(Hillshire Farm):							
Hot Links:							
Beef	C						
Regular	C						
(Hormel):							
Brown 'n Serve Sausage							
Midget Links, Pork Sausage							
(Jones):							
Brown & Serve	C					S	W
Light Breakfast Links							
(Oscar Mayer):							
Little Friers Pork	C						
SAUSAGE, POLISH (see **KIELBASA**)							
SAUSAGE, SMOKED (See **SMOKED FRANKFURTERS & SMOKED SAUSAGE**)							
SCRAPPLE:							
(Jones) Country Style	C						W
(Parks)	C					S	W

Food Item	CORN	EGGS	MILK	NUTS	PEANUT	SOY	WHEAT
SEAFOOD ENTRÉES, frozen (see also **FISH, ENTRÉES, FROZEN):**							
(Armour) *Dinner Classics,* frozen meals:							
Seafood Newburg	C	E	M		P	S	W
SEASONING MIX:							
(French's):							
Chili-O							W
Sloppy Joes							W
Spice Your Rice:							
Beef 'n Onions	C		M		P	S	W
Chicken 'n Herb	C		M		P	S	
(Kikkoman):							
Chow Mein	C		M			S	W
Fried Rice	C		M			S	W
Meat Marinade	C		M			S	W
Stir-Fry	C		M			S	W
Sweet & Sour	C					S	W
Teriyaki	C		M			S	W
SEASONINGS:							
(Ener-G Foods):							
All-Purpose	C						
All-Purpose with Lemon	C						
Herb							
Salad	C		M				
(Health Valley Foods) *Instead of Salt:*							
All Purpose							
Chicken							
Fish							
Steak & Hamburgers							
Vegetables							
Longhorn Grill Seasoning (Bernard):							
Cajun Creole							
Herbal Mesquite	C					S	W
Jalapeño	C						W
Low Salt Mesquite	C		M			S	W
Original Mesquite	C		M			S	W
Tex Mex	C						W
Mrs. Dash:							
Extra Spicy	C						
Lemon & Herb	C						

Food Item	CORN	EGGS	MILK	NUTS	PEANUT	SOY	WHEAT
Low Pepper, No Garlic	C						
Regular	C						
SEAWEED:							
(Premier Japan) Seaweeds and sea vegetable products:							
Agar-Agar Flakes							
Chopped Kombu							
Hijiki							
Instant Wakame							
Toasted Sushi Nori							
SESAME BUTTER (Erewhon)							
SESAME OIL:							
(Premier Japan), Toasted							
SESAME SEEDS:							
(Premier Japan):							
Goma Furikake, Black (Roasted)							
Goma Shio, White							
SESAME TAHINI (Erewhon)							
SHAKE MIXES:							
Artificially sweetened:							
Diet-Trim (Bernard):							
Chocolate	C		M				W
Vanilla	C		M				W
Regular (Concord):							
Banana	C		M			S	
Bananaberry	C		M			S	
Choconana	C		M			S	
Orange	C		M			S	
Pineapple	C		M			S	
Shapely Shake (Bernard):							
Chocolate	C		M			S	W
Vanilla	C		M			S	W
SHERBET:							
(Flav-O-Rich):							
Lime	C		M		P	S	W
Orange	C		M		P	S	W
Pineapple	C		M		P	S	W
Rainbow	C		M		P	S	W
Raspberry	C		M		P	S	
Vanilla Orange	C		M		P	S	W
Push-Ups (Flav-O-Rich) Orange	C		M		P	S	

Food Item	CORN	EGGS	MILK	NUTS	PEANUT	SOY	WHEAT
(Welsh Farms) Raspberry	C		M		P	S	
SHORTENING:							
Crisco:							
Butter Flavor			M			S	W
Regular						S	W
(Ener-G Foods):							
Soy-free Shortening							
SHRIMP, FROZEN:							
(Carnation):							
Hand Breaded	C		M		P	S	W
Shrimp Crisps	C	E	M		P	S	W
SLOPPY JOES, CANNED:							
(Hormel)	C					S	W
SLOPPY JOE, MIX (Tempo)	C		M			S	W
SMOKED FRANKFURTERS &							
SMOKED SAUSAGE:							
(Hillshire Farm):							
Smoked Sausage:							
Beef	C					S	W
Hot	C						
Original	C					S	W
(Hormel):							
Beef Wranglers Smoked Franks	C						
Skinless Smoked Sausage			M			S	
Smoked Pork Sausage (no link)							
Smokies:							
Cheezers Smoked Sausage	C		M				
Smoked Sausage	C						W
Wranglers (Range) Smoked Franks	C						
(Louis Rich):							
Turkey Smoked Sausage	C						
(Oscar Mayer):							
Beef Smokies	C					S	
Cheese Smokies	C		M			S	
Little Smokies	C					S	
Smokie Links	C					S	
SNACKS, PUFFS, CHIPS, CURLS:							
(Bachman):							
Bar-b-que Corn Chips	C				P	S	W
Corn Chips	C				P	S	

Food Item	CORN	EGGS	MILK	NUTS	PEANUT	SOY	WHEAT
Jax:							
Baked	C		M			S	W
Crunchy	C		M			S	W
Nacho Tortilla Chips	C		M		P	S	W
Tortilla Chips	C				P	S	
(Charles):							
Bar-B-Q Corn Chips	C		M		P	S	W
Cheese Twists	C		M		P	S	
Corn Chips	C					S	
Fried Twists	C		M		P	S	W
Nacho Tostadas	C		M		P		W
Combos (Snack Master):							
Cheese-filled Crackers	C		M		P	S	W
Cheddar Cheese	C	E	M		P	S	W
Cheese Crackers	C		M		P	S	W
Nacho Cheese	C	E	M		P	S	W
Pizza Cheese	C	E	M		P	S	W
(Eagle):							
Cantina Tortilla Chips	C		M		P	S	W
Cheese Crunch	C		M		P	S	W
(Edward & Sons):							
Crunchy Crackerballs					P	S	W
Snack Sacks:							
Sea Vegie Chips	C						W
Vegie Chips	C						W
(Frito-Lay):							
Cheddar Valley Cheese Snacks	C		M		P	S	
Cheetos, cheese snacks:							
Crunchy	C		M		P	S	
Puffed	C		M		P	S	W
Doritos	C		M		P	S	W
Fritos Corn Chips	C				P	S	
Ruffles Potato Chips	C				P	S	
(Health Valley Foods):							
Buenitos:							
Nacho Cheese & Chili	C		M				
Regular	C						
Unsalted	C						
Cheddar Lites:							
Regular	C		M				
Unsalted	C		M				

Food Item	CORN	EGGS	MILK	NUTS	PEANUT	SOY	WHEAT
Corn Chips:							
Regular	C						
Unsalted	C						
With Cheese	C		M				
Yogurt	C		M				
Tortilla Strips:							
Cheese	C		M				
Regular	C						
12 Vegetable	C						
Yogurt & Green Onion	C		M				
(Old El Paso) Nachips	C					S	
(Planters):							
Cheez Curls	C		M			S	W
Corn Chips	C					S	
Pretzels							W
Tortilla Chips:							
Nacho	C		M			S	W
Traditional	C					S	
(Snyder's of Hanover):							
Barbe'q Corn Chips	C					S	W
Cheese Twists	C		M			S	W
Mini Pretzels						S	W
Nacho Cheese Tortilla Chips	C		M			S	W
Potato Chips							
(Tio Sancho) Nacho Chips	C					S	
(Utz's):							
BBQ Corn Chips	C					S	W
Corn Chips	C						
Nacho Cheese Tortilla Chips	C		M			S	W
Tortilla Chips	C						
(Walnut Acres):							
Munchy Mix					P		
Original Snacks				N			
Tropical Mix				N			
(Wise):							
Bravos	C		M			S	W
Cheez Doodles	C		M			S	
Dipsy Doodles	C					S	

SOFT DRINKS, dietetic, artificially
sweetened:

Food Item	CORN	EGGS	MILK	NUTS	PEANUT	SOY	WHEAT
(Diet Shasta):							
Birch Beer	C		M				W
Black Cherry	C						
Caffeine-free Cola	C		M				W
Cherry Cola	C		M				W
Chocolate	C		M				W
Cola	C		M				W
Creme	C		M				W
Frolic	C					S	
Ginger Ale	C						
Grape	C						
Grapefruit	C				P	S	
Lemon Lime	C						
Orange	C					S	
Red Pop	C		M				W
Root Beer	C		M				W
Strawberry	C						
SOFT DRINKS, regular, sweetened:							
Cola, caffeine-free:							
Coke	C		M				W
Pepsi Free	C		M				W
Cola, regular:							
Pepsi	C		M				W
Creme (Adirondack)	C		M				W
Dr Pepper	C		M				W
Ginger Ale (Schweppes)	C		M				W
(Health Valley Foods):							
Apple	C						
Cola	C						
Ginger Ale	C						
Ginseng Root Beer	C						
Grape	C						
Lemon-Lime	C						
Mandarin-Lime	C						
Root Beer	C						
Sarsaparilla	C						
Wild Berry	C						
Naturale 90:							
Raspberry	C						
Root Beer:							
A & W	C		M				W

Food Item	CORN	EGGS	MILK	NUTS	PEANUT	SOY	WHEAT
Ramblin	C		M				W
Seagram's:							
Tonic Water	C						
Seltzer:							
(Manischewitz)							
(Seagram's):							
Orange							
(Vintage):							
Mandarin Orange							
Original							
Shasta:							
Black Cherry	C						
Cherry Cola	C						
Club Soda							
Shasta-free Cola, no caffeine	C		M				W
Citrus Mist	C				P	S	
Cola	C		M				W
Creme	C		M				W
Dr. Diablo	C		M				W
Ginger Ale	C		M				W
Grape	C						
Lemon Lime	C						
Orange	C				P	S	
Red Berry	C						
Red Pop	C						
Root Beer	C		M				W
Strawberry	C						
Tonic	C						
Slice:							
Lemon-Lime	C						
(Snapple):							
Creme d' Chocolate	C						
Creme d' Vanilla	C						
French Cherry	C						
Montreal Ginger Ale	C						
Orange Brite	C						
Passion Supreme	C						
Seltzer							
Wild Cranberry	C						
(Spree):							
Cherry Lime	C						

Food Item	CORN	EGGS	MILK	NUTS	PEANUT	SOY	WHEAT
Cola	C		M				W
Ginger Ale	C		M				W
Grapefruit	C						
Lemon Lime	C						
Lemon Tangerine	C						
Mandarin Lime	C						
Root Beer	C						
Tropical Blend	C						
Summer Song (Lakewood):							
Apple Berry Berry							
Ginger Ale							
Root Beer							
Sparkling Cherry							
Sparking Lemon Lime							
Sunkist Orange	C				P	S	W
Tonic Water:							
(Schweppes)	C						
(Welch's) Strawberry	C						
SORBET ((See also **FRUIT SORBET**)):							
(Le Sorbet) Raspberry							
SORELL RIDGE, Conserves							
(See **JAMS/JELLIES**)							
SOUP, canned:							
(Campbell's):							
Condensed:							
Bean with Bacon	C					S	W
Chicken & Stars	C					S	W
Chicken Barley	C		M			S	W
Chicken Noodle	C	E	M		P	S	W
Chicken Broth & Rice	C					S	W
Chicken Noodle, Homestyle	C	E	M		P	S	W
Chicken Vegetable	C	E	M		P	S	W
Chicken with Rice	C		M		P	S	W
Clam Chowder, New England	C					S	W
Cream of Mushroom	C		M			S	W
Creamy Chicken Mushroom	C		M		P	S	
Creamy Natural:							
Asparagus	C		M				W
Broccoli	C	E	M				W
Potato	C		M				W
Spinach	C		M				W

Food Item	CORN	EGGS	MILK	NUTS	PEANUT	SOY	WHEAT
French Onion	C		M			S	W
Golden Mushroom	C					S	W
Oyster Stew	C		M			S	W
Pepper Pot	C		M		P	S	W
Vegetarian Vegetable	C					S	W
Zesty Tomato	C						W
Golden Classic:							
Chicken Vegetable	C					S	W
Creamy Spinach	C		M				W
Low-sodium:							
Chicken with Noodles		E					W
Cream of Mushroom	C		M			S	W
Ready-to-Serve, *Chunky Soup:*							
Chicken Rice	C					S	W
Clam Chowder, Manhattan-style	C					S	W
New England Clam Chowder	C		M			S	W
Sirloin Burger	C		M		P	S	W
Vegetable Beef, low-sodium	C		M		P	S	
Ready-to-Serve, *Home Cookin':*							
Country Vegetable	C					S	W
Split Pea with Ham	C						
Chicken Broth:							
College Inn	C					S	W
(Swanson)	C					S	W
(Health Valley Foods):							
Vegetable Beef	C						W
Vegetable Chicken	C						W
(Pepperidge Farm):							
New England Clam Chowder	C		M			S	W
(Progresso), ready-to-serve:							
Chicken Rice	C					S	W
Chicken Vegetable	C					S	W
Lentil						S	
Lentil with Sausage	C					S	
(Walnut Acres):							
Beef Gumbo			M			S	
Beef Noodle							W
Black Bean							
Canadian Pea							W
Chicken Corn	C		M				W

Food Item	CORN	EGGS	MILK	NUTS	PEANUT	SOY	WHEAT
Chicken Curry							W
Chicken Gumbo							
Chicken Rice							W
Clambake Chowder	C		M				W
Clam Chowder:							
Manhattan							W
New England			M				W
Corn Chowder	C		M				W
Cream of Carrot			M				W
Cream of Celery			M				W
Cream of Chives			M				W
Cream of Pea			M				W
Cream of Potato			M				W
Cream of Watercress			M				W
Fish Chowder			M				W
French Onion			M			S	W
Lentil							W
Lentil with Hot Dogs	C		M				W
Navy Bean			M			S	W
Scotch Broth			M				W
Tomato			M				W
Tomato Beef Consomme							
Tomato Rice			M				W
Vegetable Beef						S	W
Vegetarian Vegetable	C					S	W
Frozen:							
(Myers) *Super Bell:*							
Bean & Ham	C	E				S	W
Chicken Corn	C					S	W
Chicken Noodle	C					S	W
Clam Chowder, New England	C	E	M		P	S	W
Cream of Broccoli	C	E	M		P	S	W
Cream of Mushroom	C	E	M		P	S	W
Cream of Potato	C	E	M		P	S	W
Seafood Bisque	C	E	M		P	S	W
Split Pea & Ham	C					S	W
Vegetable Beef	C		M			S	W
SOUP MIX, instant:							
(Kikkoman):							
Aka Miso	C					S	W

Food Item	CORN	EGGS	MILK	NUTS	PEANUT	SOY	WHEAT
Egg Flower Soup:							
Corn	C		M			S	W
Hot & Sour	C		M			S	W
Shrimp	C					S	W
Vegetable	C		M			S	W
Osuimono	C					S	W
Shiro Miso	C					S	W
Tofu Miso	C					S	W
Wakame (seaweed)	C					S	W
(Lipton):							
Cup-A-Soup:							
Chicken	C	E				S	W
Chicken Vegetable, with White							
Meat	C	E				S	W
Cream of Chicken	C		M		P	S	W
Creamy Chicken Vegetable	C				P	S	W
Garden Vegetable	C	E				S	W
Virginia Pea	C					S	W
Cup-A-Soup *Trim*:							
French Onion	C		M			S	W
Med-Diet (Ener-G Foods), gluten-free,							
wheat-free instant soups:							
Cream of Mushroom	C		M			S	
Tomato	C						
SOUP MIX, regular:							
(Campbell):							
Noodle	C	E				S	W
(Edward & Sons) (*Miso-Cup*):							
Original						S	
Seaweed						S	
(Fearn):							
Lentil Minestrone	C	E	M		P	S	W
Split Pea	C	E	M		P	S	
(Knorr) Beefy Vegetable	C		M		P	S	W
(Lipton):							
Country Vegetable	C		M			S	W
Cream of Mushroom à la Reine	C		M				W
Creamy Herb	C		M				W
Hearty Chicken Noodle	C	E				S	W
Hearty Minestrone	C		M			S	W
Hearty Noodle	C	E				S	W

Food Item	CORN	EGGS	MILK	NUTS	PEANUT	SOY	WHEAT
Onion	C		M			S	W
(Manischewitz):							
Minestrone	C					S	W
Split Pea	C					S	W
Vegetable		E					W
(Mrs. Grass):							
Homestyle Chickeny Noodle	C	E			P	S	W
Onion	C		M			S	W
(Walnut Acres):							
Beef Barley	C				P	S	W
Chicken Mushroom	C				P	S	W
Chicken Noodle	C	E			P	S	W
Cream of Mushroom			M				
Lentil							
Minestrone						S	W
Split Pea & Barley						S	
Tomato-Vegetable	C						W
Wild Rice & Split Pea	C				P	S	W
SOUR CREAM:							
(Flav-O-Rich)			M				
SOY MILK POWDER:							
(Ener-G Foods) SoyQuik						S	
SOY PRODUCTS:							
(Fearn):							
Soya Granules						S	
Soya Powder						S	
Soya Protein Isolate						S	
Soy-O Cereal						S	W
(Health Valley Foods):							
Soy Moo, beverage:							
Carob						S	
Plain						S	
Tamari-ya Soy Sauce						S	
Tofu-Ya Tofu						S	
SOY SAUCE (See **SAUCE**)							
SPAGHETTI (See **PASTA**)							
SPAGHETTI SAUCE, jarred:							
(Aunt Millie's) meatless			M		P		
(County Cuisine), low sodium	C					S	
(Enrico's):							
Homemade Style							

Food Item	CORN	EGGS	MILK	NUTS	PEANUT	SOY	WHEAT
Marinara						S	
No-salt Added							
With Mushrooms							
With Mushrooms, Green Peppers							
(Ferrara) Pasta Sauce:							
Bolognese						S	
Neopolitan						S	
Sicilian						S	
(Francesco Rinaldi):							
Marinara	C					S	
Meat-flavored	C		M			S	
Meatless	C		M			S	
No-Salt			M			S	
With mushrooms	C		M			S	
(Progresso):							
Carbonara	C		M				W
Marinara			M			S	
(Ragu):							
Chunky Gardenstyle:							
With Green & Red Peppers	C		M			S	
With Tomatoes, Garlic, Onions	C		M			S	
Homestyle						S	
Marinara	C					S	
SPAM:							
Deviled *Spam*						S	W
Spam							
Spam, smoke flavored	C						W
Spam with Cheese Chunks			M				
SPICE YOUR RICE							
(See **SEASONING MIX**)							
SPINACH, frozen:							
(Stouffer's):							
Spinach Souffle		E	M		P		W
SQUID, frozen:							
Golden Squid Rings (Goya)	C				P	S	W
STEAK SAUCE (See also **SAUCE,**							
prepared):							
(French's)	C						W
Heinz 57	C		M			S	W
STIR-FRY MIX (Concord)	C		M			S	W

Food Item	CORN	EGGS	MILK	NUTS	PEANUT	SOY	WHEAT
STOUFFER'S:							
Entrées:							
Chicken Pie	C	E	M				W
Creamed Chicken	C		M				W
Creamed Chipped Beef	C		M				W
Escalloped Chicken & Noodles	C	E	M				W
Macaroni & Cheese	C	E	M		P		W
Tuna Noodle Casserole	C	E	M		P		W
Turkey Pie	C	E	M				W
Lean Cuisine:							
Cheese Cannelloni	C	E	M		P		W
Chicken Cacciatore	C	E	M		P		W
Chicken & Vegetables	C	E	M				W
Veal Lasagna	C		M			S	W
Side Dishes:							
Escalloped Apples	C		M		P		W
Fettucini Primavera	C	E	M		P		W
Linguine with Pesto Sauce	C		M	N	P		W
Noodles Romanoff	C	E	M		P		W
Scalloped Potatoes	C		M		P		W
Spinach Souffle		E	M		P		W
Yams & Apples	C						W
STUFFED PEPPERS, frozen:							
(Health Valley Foods) *Meals For Two:*							
Stuffed Peppers			M			S	W
STUFFING MIX:							
Chicken:							
Rice-a-Roni	C		M			S	W
Stove Top	C		M			S	W
SUGAR SUBSTITUTE:							
Equal:							
Packets	C						
Tablets	C		M				
Sugar Twin:							
Brown Sugar Replacement	C		M				W
White Sugar Replacement	C						W
Packets	C						
SUMMER SAUSAGE:							
(Hormel):							
Beefy Summer Sausage			M				

Food Item	CORN	EGGS	MILK	NUTS	PEANUT	SOY	WHEAT
Lumberjack Beef Summer Sausage			M				W
Sliced Beef Summer Sausage			M				
Tangy Summer Sausage			M				
SUNFLOWER BUTTER (Erewhon)							
SYRUP:							
Chocolate:							
(Hershey's)	C				P	S	
Quik	C						
Karo:							
Dark	C						
Light	C						
Pancake	C						
(Ferrara):							
Amarena (wild cherry)	C						
Granatina (grenadine)	C						
Lampone (raspberry)	C						
Menta (mint)							
Orzata (almond)				N			
Tamarindo (tamarind)	C		M				W
(Knott's Berry Farm):							
Boysenberry	C						
Strawberry	C						
Pancake or Waffle:							
Aunt Jemima:							
Butter Lite	C		M				W
Lite	C		M				W
Regular	C		M				W
Country Syrup (Knott's)	C		M				W
Mrs. Butterworth's, lite	C		M				W

Food Item	CORN	EGGS	MILK	NUTS	PEANUT	SOY	WHEAT

T

TABOULI:
  (Fantastic) mix

| | | | | | | | W |

TACO BELL:

Corn Tortilla	C						
Flour Tortilla	C				P	S	W
Red Sauce	C					S	W

TACO SEASONING MIX:

(McCormick)	C		M			S	W
(Old El Paso)	C						
(Ortega)	C		M				W
(Tio Sancho)	C		M			S	W

TACO SAUCE:

| (Old El Paso), hot | C | | | | | | W |

TACO SHELLS:

| (Old El Paso) | C | | | | | S | |
| (Tio Sancho) | C | | | | | S | |

TAMALES, canned:
  (Old El Paso):

| Tamales | C | | | | | | W |
| Tamales with Chili Gravy | C | | | | | | W |

TAMARI:
  (Erewhon):

| Shoyu Tamari | | | | | | S | W |

TAPIOCA FLOUR:
  (Ener-G Foods) Tapioca Flour

TEA:
  (Bigelow):
    Cinnamon Stick
    Constant Comment
    Earl Grey
    English Teatime
    Lemon Lift
    Plantation Mint
    Raspberry Royale

Food Item	CORN	EGGS	MILK	NUTS	PEANUT	SOY	WHEAT
TEA, HERBAL:							
(Bigelow)							
Almond Orange				N			
Apple & Spice							W
Apple Orchard							
Chamomile Mint							
Cinnamon Orange							W
Feeling Free							
Fruit & Almond				N			
Hibiscus & Rose Hips							
I Love Lemon							
Lemon & C	C						
Looking Good							
Mint Blend							
Mint Medley							
Nice Over Ice							
Orange & C	C						
Orange & Spice							
Roasted Grains & Carob							W
Sweet Dreams							
Take-A-Break							W
(Celestial Seasonings)							
Almond Sunset				N			W
Chamomile							
Cinnamon Apple Spice							W
Cinnamon Rose							W
Cranberry Cove							
Diet Partner							
Emperor's Choice							
Ginseng Plus							W
Grandma's Tummy Mint							
Island Orange							
Lemon Iced Delight							
Lemon Mist	C						
Lemon Zinger	C						
Mandarin Orange Spice							
Mellow Mint							
Morning Thunder							
Mo's 24	C						
Peppermint							

Food Item	CORN	EGGS	MILK	NUTS	PEANUT	SOY	WHEAT
Raspberry Patch							
Red Zinger	C						
Rosehips							
Rostaroma Grain & Spice							W
Sleepytime							
Spearmint							
Sunburst C	C						
(Health Valley Foods):							
Lively Daytime							
Tranquil Evening							
Zesty Morning							
(Lipton):							
Flavored Tea:							
Amaretto				N			
Cherry Almond				N			
Cinnamon							
Orange & Spice							
Herbal:							
Almond Pleasure	C			N			W
Berry Blush							
Cinnamon Apple							
Gentle Orange							
Ginger Twist							
Lemon Soother	C						
Quietly Chamomile							
TEA, ICED:							
Mix:							
(4 C) Sugar & Lemon-Flavored	C						W
(Tetley) Iced Tea Mix	C						W
Refrigerated, Dairy-Pak:							
(Flav-O-Rich) *Nestea*	C						
TEA, JAPANESE:							
(Erewhon):							
Mu #9							
Mu #16							
(Premier Japan):							
Bancha							
Genmaicha							
Kukicha							
TEMPURA:							
Batter, mix:							

Food Item	CORN	EGGS	MILK	NUTS	PEANUT	SOY	WHEAT
(Fantastic)	C					S	W
THURINGER:							
(Hormel):							
Old Smokehouse Thuringer			M				
Sliced Buffet Thuringer			M			S	W
Sliced *Old Smokehouse* Thuringer			M				
TOASTER CAKE/PASTRY:							
(Freihofer's) Corn Toasties	C	E	M		P	S	W
Pop-Tarts (Kellogg's):							
Frosted Strawberry	C		M			S	W
Toast-r-Cake (Thomas'):							
Blueberry	C	E	M			S	W
Bran	C	E	M			S	W
Corn	C	E	M			S	W
Toastettes (Nabisco):							
Frosted:							
Brown Sugar Cinnamon	C		M			S	W
Fudge	C		M			S	W
Strawberry	C		M			S	W
Regular:							
Apple	C		M			S	W
Blueberry	C		M			S	W
Cherry	C		M			S	W
Strawberry	C		M			S	W
TOFU, refrigerated:							
(Tomsun)						S	
TOFU MIXES:							
(Fantastic)							
Burger Mix	C					S	W
Tofu Scrambler	C					S	W
TOMATO SAUCE, canned:							
(Del Monte):							
No-Salt							
Regular	C						
(Health Valley Foods):							
No-Salt							
Pasta Sauce, *Bellissimo*			M				
Regular						S	W
TOMATOES, canned:							
Italian (Ferrara)							

Food Item	CORN	EGGS	MILK	NUTS	PEANUT	SOY	WHEAT
(Old El Paso):							
Tomatoes & Green Chilies							
Tomatoes & Jalapeños							
Whole (Redpack), with Puree	C						
TOPPINGS:							
(Raffetto):							
Cream:							
Butterscotch Brandy Cream	C		M			S	W
Coconut Rum Cream	C	E	M		P	S	
Fruit:							
Nesselro Fruit	C		M	N			W
Peach Brandy Fruit							
Sauce Melba, Raspberry	C						
Twin Berry Kirsh Fruit							
Fudge:							
Café Kahlua Fudge	C		M			S	W
Creme de Menthe Fudge	C		M			S	W
Grand Marnier Fudge	C		M			S	W
Hazelnut Amoretto Fudge	C		M	N		S	W
Irish Cream Fudge	C		M			S	W
Walnut Crunch Fudge	C		M	N		S	
(Smucker's):							
Butterscotch	C	E	M		P	S	W
Caramel	C	E	M		P	S	W
Chocolate Fudge	C	E	M		P	S	W
Hot Fudge	C	E	M		P	S	
Magic Shell:							
Chocolate	C	E			P	S	
Chocolate Fudge	C	E	M		P	S	
Strawberry	C						
Walnuts in Syrup	C			N			
TORTILLAS:							
(Baja) Flour, refrigerated	C					S	W
(Health Valley Foods), *Corntillas*	C						
(Old El Paso), canned	C						
TORTILLA CHIPS (See **SNACKS**)							
TOSTADA SHELLS:							
(Old El Paso)	C					S	
TRAIL MIX:							
(Walnut Acres)				N			

Food Item	CORN	EGGS	MILK	NUTS	PEANUT	SOY	WHEAT
TROPICANA (see **FRUIT DRINKS** and **FRUIT JUICES**)							
TUNA, canned:							
(Bumble Bee):							
Chunk White, in Oil	C					S	W
Solid White:							
In Oil	C					S	W
In Water	C					S	W
(Health Valley Foods):							
Chunk Light	C					S	
No Salt	C					S	
TUNA, ENTRÉES, frozen:							
(Stouffer's):							
Tuna Noodle Casserole	C	E	M		P		W
TURKEY, canned:							
(Hormel) Chunk Turkey			M				
TURKEY, fresh:							
(Louis Rich):							
Ground Turkey							
Turkey Breakfast Sausage							
Turkey Breast							
Turkey Breast Slices							
Turkey Breast Tenderloins							
Turkey Drumsticks							
Turkey Thigh							
Turkey Wing							
Turkey Wing Drumettes							
Whole Turkey							
Mr. Turkey, ground							
(Turkey Store) ground							
TURKEY, frozen:							
(Banquet) Turkey Dinner	C		M		P	S	W
(Myers) Turkey Pie	C		M		P	S	W
(Stouffer's):							
Turkey Pie	C	E	M				W
(Weight Watchers) Stuffed Breast	C		M		P	S	W
TURKEY, prepared:							
(Bil Mar):							
Breast of Turkey							
Mr. Turkey:							
Breast, Deli-pack and Chubs:							

Food Item	CORN	EGGS	MILK	NUTS	PEANUT	SOY	WHEAT
Barbecued	C						
Smoked	C					S	W
Frankfurters:							
Cheese Franks	C		M				
Franks	C						
Ground Turkey							
Lunch Meats:							
Bologna	C						
Chopped Ham	C					S	W
Cotto Salami	C					S	W
Pastrami	C						
Red Rind Bologna	C						
Smoked Ham	C					S	W
Smoked Turkey	C						
Smoked Turkey Breast	C					S	W
Spiced Luncheon Loaf	C						
Turkey Breast							
(De Witt's Table Ready Meats):							
Barbecue Turkey Breast							
Oven Roasted Turkey Breast							
Smoked Turkey Breast	C						
Louis Rich:							
Franks/Smoked Sausage:							
Turkey Cheese Franks	C		M				
Turkey Franks	C						
Turkey Smoked Sausage	C						
Sliced Meats:							
Oven Roasted Turkey Breast							
Oven Roasted Chicken Breast			M				
Smoked Turkey							
Smoked Turkey Breast							
Turkey Bologna	C						
Turkey Cotto Salami							
Turkey Ham							
Turkey Ham, Chopped							
Turkey Luncheon Loaf							
Turkey Pastrami							
Turkey Salami							
Turkey Summer Sausage	C		M				
TURNOVERS, frozen:							
(Pepperidge Farm) Raspberry	C	E	M		P	S	W
TWINKIES	C	E	M		P	S	W

Food Item	CORN	EGGS	MILK	NUTS	PEANUT	SOY	WHEAT

V

VAN DE KAMP'S (see **FISH**)

VEAL ENTRÉES, frozen:
  (Stouffer's):
    Lean Cuisine:
      Veal Lasagna

VEGETABLE CRISP (Ore-Ida):
  Broccoli
  Cauliflower
  Medley
  Mushrooms
  Zucchini

VEGETABLES, frozen:
  (Ore-Ida):
    Cob Corn
    Stew Vegetables

VEGETABLE SALAD:
  (Hanover) Deli-Style

VEGETARIAN MIXES:
  (Fearn):
    Bean Barley Stew
    Blackbean Creole Mix
    Breakfast Patty Mix
    Burger Mixes:
      Brazil Nut
      Sesame
      Sunflower
    Falafel
    Tri-Bean Casserole
    Nature's Burger, mix
  (Walnut Acres):
    Falafel

VIENNA SAUSAGE, canned:
  (Hormel):
    Chicken Vienna Sausage
    Vienna Sausage

Food Item	CORN	EGGS	MILK	NUTS	PEANUT	SOY	WHEAT
Veal Lasagna	C		M			S	W
Broccoli	C	E	M			S	W
Cauliflower	C	E	M			S	W
Medley	C	E	M			S	W
Mushrooms	C	E	M			S	W
Zucchini	C	E	M			S	W
Cob Corn	C						
Stew Vegetables							
(Hanover) Deli-Style	C						W
Bean Barley Stew	C	E	M		P	S	W
Blackbean Creole Mix	C	E	M		P	S	
Breakfast Patty Mix						S	W
Brazil Nut				N	P	S	W
Sesame						S	W
Sunflower					P	S	W
Falafel						S	
Tri-Bean Casserole	C	E	M		P	S	
Nature's Burger, mix					P	S	W
Falafel	C						
Chicken Vienna Sausage	C		M			S	W
Vienna Sausage	C		M				

Food Item	CORN	EGGS	MILK	NUTS	PEANUT	SOY	WHEAT

W

WAFFLES:
  Frozen:
    (Downyflake):

Food Item	CORN	EGGS	MILK	NUTS	PEANUT	SOY	WHEAT
Buttermilk	C	E	M			S	W
Regular	C	E	M			S	W

    (Eggo):

Food Item	CORN	EGGS	MILK	NUTS	PEANUT	SOY	WHEAT
Buttermilk		E	M			S	W
Homestyle		E	M			S	W
Nutri•Grain, Raisin Bran		E	M			S	W

WALNUT ACRES:
  Baking Powder

Food Item	CORN	EGGS	MILK	NUTS	PEANUT	SOY	WHEAT
Baking Powder	C		M				

  Breads:

Food Item	CORN	EGGS	MILK	NUTS	PEANUT	SOY	WHEAT
Cornell Formula	C	E	M			S	W
Molasses Bran	C						W
Oatmeal Hearth	C	E					W
Raisin	C		M				W
Raisin Bran	C						W
Rye	C		M				W
Soya Carob			M			S	W
12-Grain	C	E				S	W
Whole Wheat	C		M				W

  Bread Mixes:

Food Item	CORN	EGGS	MILK	NUTS	PEANUT	SOY	WHEAT
Apricot Nut	C		M	N		S	W
Banana Nut	C		M	N		S	W
Date Nut	C		M	N		S	W
High Lysine Corn	C		M				W
Spicy Apple Nut	C		M	N		S	W
Wheat-free Raisin Cinnamon	C		M			S	W

  Cakes:

Food Item	CORN	EGGS	MILK	NUTS	PEANUT	SOY	WHEAT
Apricot Nut		E	M	N			W
Fruitcake	C	E	M	N			W

  Condiments:

Food Item	CORN	EGGS	MILK	NUTS	PEANUT	SOY	WHEAT
Barbecue Sauce	C						W

    Ketchup:

Food Item	CORN	EGGS	MILK	NUTS	PEANUT	SOY	WHEAT
Salted	C						W

Food Item	CORN	EGGS	MILK	NUTS	PEANUT	SOY	WHEAT
Unsalted	C						W
Gelatin							
Meat & Chicken Products:							
Beans & Hot Dogs							
Beef Stew			M				W
Braised Beef Hash							
Chicken Stew			M				W
Chili Con Carne	C						
Noodles & Ground Beef			M			S	W
Muffin Mixes:							
Blueberry	C		M			S	W
Bran	C		M				W
Corn	C		M			S	W
Maple Granola	C		M	N	P	S	W
Pancake Mixes:							
Buckwheat	C		M				W
Buttermilk Johnny Cake	C		M			S	
Hi-Bran	C		M			S	W
Rice	C					S	
12 Grain	C		M			S	W
Unbleached White with Soy	C		M			S	W
Wheatless	C		M			S	W
Whole Wheat with Soy	C		M			S	W
Pasta:							
Corn:							
Elbows	C						
Spaghetti	C						
Vegetable Elbow Macaroni							W
Whole Wheat:							
Egg Noodles		E					W
Elbow Macaroni							W
Sesame Spirals							W
Spaghetti							W
Pasta Sauces:							
Clam							W
Marinara			M			S	W
Spaghetti			M				W
Rice & Grain Mixes:							
Amaranth Medley							W
Bombay Rice					P		

Food Item	CORN	EGGS	MILK	NUTS	PEANUT	SOY	WHEAT
Herbed Bulgur Rice				N			W
Near East Kasha							W
Oriental Rice						S	
Red Beans and Rice							
Rice Pilaf						S	
Savory Millet						S	W
Spanish Rice							
Sustains							W
Three-Grain Rice Blend							
Salts & Seasonings:							
Hickory Flavor Bakon Yeast							
Kelp Granules							
Kome Miso						S	
Orsa Natural Mineral Salt							
Tamari Soy Sauce						S	W
Vegetable Seasoning							
Vegetarian Mixes:							
Falafel	C						
Vanilla Bean							
Vanilla Extract	C						W
WATER ICE (See FROZEN DESSERTS & CONFECTIONS)							
WEIGHT WATCHERS:							
Apple Snack							
Margarine, Reduced Calorie:							
Soft	C	E			P	S	
Soft, unsalted	C	E			P	S	
Sticks	C				P	S	
Mayonnaise:							
Low Sodium	C	E				S	W
Regular	C	E				S	W
Nutri-Treat:							
Chocolate	C		M		P	S	
Eggnog	C		M				
Strawberry	C		M				
Vanilla Marshmallow	C		M				
Salad Dressing	C	E				S	W
Thousand Island Dressing	C	E				S	W
WELCH'S:							
Canned & Bottled Juices:							

Food Item	C O R N	E G G S	M I L K	N U T S	P E A N U T	S O Y	W H E A T
Orchard Apple-Grape							
Orchard Harvest Blend							
Orchard North Country Blend							
Orchard Vineyard Blend							
Purple Grape	C						
Red Grape	C						
Sparkling Red Grape							
Sparkling White Grape							
Tomato							
White Grape	C						
Frozen Concentrates:							
Cranberry-Apple Juice Cocktail	C						
Cranberry-Grape Juice Cocktail	C						
Cranberry Juice Cocktail	C						
Orchard Apple-Grape							
Orchard Grape Juice							
Orchard Harvest Blend							
Orchard North Country Blend							
Sweetened Grape Juice	C						
Fruit Drinks:							
Grape Juice Beverage	C						
Welchade Grape Drink	C						
WHEAT:							
Bulgur (Old World)							
WHEAT GERM:							
(Fearn) Naturfresh, raw							W
(Health Valley Foods):							
Regular							W
With Almonds, Dates				N			W
With Bananas, Hawaiian Fruit							W
(Kretschmer):							
Honey Crunch	C						W
Regular							W
WHIPPED TOPPING:							
Reddi-Wip	C		M		P	S	
Nondairy:							
(Rich's):							
Rich Whip, aerosol	C				P	S	
Frozen	C		M		P	S	
Liquid	C				P	S	
WINE COOLERS:							
(Bartles & Jaymes)	C		M				W

Food Item	CORN	EGGS	MILK	NUTS	PEANUT	SOY	WHEAT
WISH-BONE (see **SALAD DRESSING**)							
WURST (See also **KNOCKWURST**):							
(Hillshire Farm):							
Cheddarwurst	C		M			S	W

Food Item	C O R N	E G G S	M I L K	N U T S	P E A N U T	S O Y	W H E A T

X

XANTHAN GUM:
  (Ener-G Foods)

	C						

Food Item	C O R N	E G G S	M I L K	N U T S	P E A N U T	S O Y	W H E A T

Y

YAMS, frozen:
  (Mrs. Paul's):

Food Item	CORN	EGGS	MILK	NUTS	PEANUT	SOY	WHEAT
Candied	C		M				W
Yams 'N Apples	C		M				W
(Stouffer's):							
Yams & Apples	C						W
YEAST:							
(Fleischmann's):							
Active Dry	C						
Compressed	C						
(Walnut Acres) Hickory Flavor							
Bakon Yeast							
YOGURT:							
(Colombo):							
Banana Strawberry	C		M				W
Blueberry	C		M				W W
Breakfast Granola	C		M	N			W W
Cherry Vanilla	C		M				W
French Vanilla			M				
Honey Vanilla			M				
Lemon			M				
Natural Lite			M				
Peach Melba	C		M				W
Piña Colada	C		M				W
Plain			M				
Raspberry	C		M				W
Strawberry	C		M				W W
Strawberry Vanilla	C		M				W W
Wildberry	C		M				W
(Dannon):							
Extra Smooth:							
Blueberry			M				
Cherry			M				
Mixed Berries			M				

Food Item	C O R N	E G G S	M I L K	N U T S	P E A N U T	S O Y	W H E A T
Peach			M				
Piña Colada			M				
Raspberry			M				
Strawberry			M				
Strawberry-Banana			M				
Lowfat:							
Banana			M				
Blueberry	C		M				
Boysenberry	C		M				
Cherry	C		M				
Coffee			M				
Dutch Apple	C		M				
Lemon			M				
Mixed Berries			M				
Peach	C		M				
Piña Colada	C		M				
Plain			M				
Raspberry	C		M				
Strawberry	C		M				
Strawberry-Banana			M				
Vanilla			M				
Mini-Pack:							
Blueberry	C		M				
Mixed Berries			M				
Raspberry	C		M				
Strawberry	C		M				
Supreme:							
Banana, Strawberries			M				
Blackberry, Raspberries			M				
Coconut, Cherries			M				
Mixed Berries, Blueberries			M				
Passion Fruit, Peaches			M				
Strawberry, Strawberry			M				
(Flavo-O-Rich) Lowfat:							
Black Cherry	C		M				W
Blueberry	C		M				W
Lemon	C		M				W
Mandarin Orange	C		M				W
Pineapple	C		M				W
Peach	C		M				W

Food Item	CORN	EGGS	MILK	NUTS	PEANUT	SOY	WHEAT
Plain	C		M				W
Strawberry	C		M				W
(Flav-O-Rich) Swiss Style:							
Black Cherry	C		M				W
Blueberry	C		M				W
Peach	C		M				W
Pineapple	C		M				W
Red Raspberry	C		M				W
Spiced Apple	C		M				W
Strawberry	C		M				W
(Golden Harvest):							
Peach	C		M				
(La Yogurt):							
Peach			M				
Vanilla			M				
(New Country):							
Peaches 'n Cream	C		M				W
(Whitney's):							
Strawberry Banana		E	M				
(Yoplait):							
Breakfast Yogurt:							
Orchard Fruits			M	N			W
Strawberry-Banana			M	N			W
Custard Style:							
Banana	C		M				
Raspberry	C		M				
Vanilla	C		M				
Original:							
Raspberry			M				
YOGURT, frozen:							
(Colombo) Soft-Serve:							
Vanilla	C	E	M				
(Tuscan Farms) Vanilla	C		M		P	S	W
***YOO-HOO* SYRUP**	C		M				

Food Item	CORN	EGGS	MILK	NUTS	PEANUT	SOY	WHEAT

Z

ZUCCHINI, frozen, prepared:

Food Item	CORN	EGGS	MILK	NUTS	PEANUT	SOY	WHEAT
(Mrs. Paul's) Zucchini Sticks	C		M			S	W

Glossary of
Food Additives and
Ingredients

You've just reached for a box containing "unbleached enriched wheat flour, nonfat milk, coconut oil, sugar, partially hydrogenated vegetable shortening, salt, onion powder, vinegar, yeast, garlic powder, mono- and diglycerides, and lecithin," and a bottle of "partially hydrogenated soybean oil, water, white distilled vinegar, salt, sugar, dried garlic, xanthan gum, polysorbate 60, artificial colors, spices, calcium disodium EDTA, and FD&C Yellow No. 5," and you're about to add these items (onion and garlic croutons and creamy Italian dressing) to your salad.

But, wait a minute. You're allergic to corn and eggs: Should you be indulging in these additive-laden delicacies? Could any of these ingredients have been derived from foods you're allergic to?

Let's take a closer look: Onion and garlic croutons contain some fairly straightforward ingredients: flour, sugar, nonfat milk, coconut oil, salt, onion powder, garlic powder, and yeast. But what exactly are mono- and diglycerides or lecithin? The creamy Italian salad dressing has a few mysterious ingredients, too: Polysorbate 60, calcium disodium EDTA, xanthan gum, and FD&C Yellow No. 5.

To help you decide which additives you might want to avoid on your particular diet, consult the following list of more than 300 ingredients. Common methods of synthesis for each ingredient have been included, as well as a code (C = corn, E = eggs, M = milk, N = nuts, P = peanuts, S = soybeans, W = wheat and gluten) to identify the food sources that may have been used. (–)

indicates that an additive probably does not contain any of the seven aforementioned allergens if prepared according to common manufacturing techniques.

Please note: An additive that rates a C for corn or a W for wheat or gluten, for example, might *not* contain any of the proteins from those substances; the list only suggests that such a possibility exists. Only you and your physician can decide how stringent your diet should be, and what foods and food additives you must avoid.

Many physicians are concerned that by avoiding too many food products an allergic person's nutrition might be compromised, but let's be honest: No one's health was ever harmed by turning down a Twinkie. There are no "cures" for food allergies—there is only *avoidance*. If you are unsure about the safety of any product, the best advice is to just say "No, thank you."

Acetic acid (ethanoic acid)—Can be produced by the fermentation of carbohydrates, by organic synthesis, by the oxidation-fermentation of ethanol, or by the destructive distillation of wood. Wood distillation was once the principal source of acetic acid in the United States, but today the three main routes of production are acetaldehyde oxidation, liquid-phase hydrocarbon oxidation, or methanol carbonylation. (–)

Aconitic acid—Can be isolated during sugarcane processing. (–)

Adipic acid—Commonly prepared by nitric acid oxidation of cyclohexanol and/or cyclohexanone. (–)

Agar-agar—Prepared from marine algae. (–)

Albumen (albumin)—Egg white. (E)

Alcohol—Can be derived from the fermentation of a starch, sugar, or carbohydrate. Any product containing alcohol may have been derived from the fermentation of grain, and even though some manufacturers believe that the gluten portion of the grain is destroyed or changed by the cooking and distillation processes, cautious individuals on strict gluten-free diets are often advised to avoid all alcoholic beverages and flavorings with an alcohol base unless certified as gluten-free. (C,W)

Alcoholic beverages:

    Absinthe—Made from brandy and aromatic flavorings such as fennel, artemisia. (–)

Aquavit—Scandinavian beverage fermented and distilled from grain or potatoes. (C,W)

Bitters—Alcoholic tonic flavored with herbs. (C,W)

Brandy—Produced from grapes, citrus, or other fruits. (–)

Chica—South American beverage traditionally made by the "chew and spit" process of fermentation, from corn, peanuts, plantain, potatoes, or other starch crops. (C,P,W)

Cider, hard—From fermented apples or other fruit. (–)

Gin—Produced by distillation from mash made from rye or other grains, or by the redistillation of distilled spirits, or from a mixture of neutral spirits with juniper and other aromatic berries. Botanical flavorings, such as anise, coriander, bitter almonds, lemon and orange peel give each brand of gin a distinctive flavor. (C,W)

Holland Gin—Derived from juniper berries and cereal grains. (C,W)

Mead—Unaged, unflavored distillate, fermented from a honey solution. (–)

Okelehao (oke)—Hawaiian distillate from molasses, rice, or dasheen (taro). (–)

Rum—Produced from fermented juice of sugarcane. (–)

Sake—Japanese beverage made from fermented rice. (–)

Tequila—Produced from fermented juice of mezcal azul cactus. (–)

Vodka—If it is produced from grain it must be treated with activated carbon or highly refined to ensure that it has no aroma or taste. (C,W)

Whiskey:

> **Canadian whisky**—Made from corn, rye, and barley malt. (C,W)

> **Irish whiskey**—A blend of grain and malt whiskeys. (C,W)

> **Rye, bourbon, and corn whiskey**—All are mixtures of rye, corn, wheat, and malted barley. (C,W)

> **Scotch whiskey**—Most brands of Scotch are blends of grain whiskeys, and malt whiskeys, which are produced by drying malted barley over a peat fire. (C,W)

Alginic acid—From brown algae. (–)

Almonds—Tree nuts, botanically related to apricots, cherries, peaches, and plums. (N)

Aluminum calcium silicate (scolecite, heulandite)—Mineral. (–)

Aluminum sodium silicate (analcite, natrolite)—Mineral. (–)

Aluminum sulfate—(–)

Ammonium chloride—Synthetic. (–)

Ammonium hydrogen carbonate—Prepared from carbon dioxide and ammonia water. (–)

Ammonium hydroxide—Synthetic. (–)

Ammonium polyphosphates—Synthetic. (–)

Ammonium sulfate—From sulfuric acid with ammonium hydroxide. (–)

Annatto (bixin, norbixin)—A yellowish-red dye obtained from seeds of the annatto tree, *Bixa orellana.* (–)

Aragum gum—Combination of gum arabic and cornstarch. (C)

Arrowroot—A nongrain starch from the roots of the tropical plant *Maranta arundinacea.* (–)

Artificial colors—Many common colors are synthetic; derived from processing coal.

Artificial flavors—Most manufacturers regard their formulas as proprietary and will not disclose the chemicals used in manufacturing.

Ascorbic acid (vitamin C)—May be manufactured by biological synthesis on a corn sugar syrup base. (C)

Aspartame—Low-calorie nutritive sweetener. (–)

Aspartic acid—Nonessential amino acid. (–)

BHA (butylated hydroxyanisole)—Synthetic antioxidant. (–)

BHT (butylated hydroxytoluene)—Synthetic antioxidant. (–)

Baking powder—Powdered mixture of baking soda, starch, and an acidic compound such as cream of tartar. Often contains cornstarch. (C)

Baking soda—Sodium bicarbonate. (–)

Barley—Cereal grain; to be avoided on a gluten-free diet. (W)

Barley malt—Sprouted barley. (W)

Beeswax—From honeycomb. (–)

Beet juice—Vegetable dye. (–)

Bentonite—From a clay deposit in the western United States. (–)

Benzoate of soda (benzoic acid)—Prepared synthetically. (–)

Benzoic acid—Manufactured from phthalic anhydride, benzotri-chloride, or toluene. (–)

Beta-amylase—Enzyme that can be derived from soybean processing. (S)

Beta-carotene—An isomer of carotene; can come from corn or be synthetically produced from acetone. Marketed as dry crystals, or as a liquid or semisolid suspension in vegetable, peanut, and butter oils. (C,M,P,S)

Blue cheese—Semisoft cow's-milk cheese with greenish-blue mold; inoculated with *Penicillium roqueforti*. (M)

Brominated vegetable oil—Combination of bromine, a halogen, with oils such as corn, peanut, and soybean. (C,P,S)

Brown sugar—Partially refined beet or cane sugar. (–)

Calcium acetate—Calcium salt of acetic acid. (–)

Calcium alginate—Calcium salt of alginic acid. (–)

Calcium carbonate—By-product of lime soda process. (–)

Calcium chloride—By-product of Solvay (ammonia-soda) process, or from salt brine. (–)

Calcium citrate—Calcium salt of citric acid. (C)

Calcium d-gluconate—Calcium salt prepared from gluconic acid. (C)

Calcium disodium EDTA (ethylenediamine tetraacetic acid)—Synthetically prepared preservative. (–)

Calcium hydroxide—From lime. (–)

Calcium lactate—Calcium salt of lactic acid. (C,M)

Calcium oxide—From limestone. (–)

Calcium polyphosphates—Synthetic. (–)

Calcium propionate—Prepared commercially from propionic acid. (–)

Calcium silicate—Mineral or synthetic. (–)

Calcium sorbate—Synthetic. (–)

Calcium stearate—Calcium salt or stearic acid. (C,P,S)

Calcium stearoyl-2-lactylate—Manufactured by the reaction of stearic acid and lactic acid; or prepared synthetically. (C,M,P,S)

Calcium sulphate (gypsum, plaster of Paris)—Mineral. (–)

Camembert cheese—Ripened by species of *Penicillium*. (M)

Candelilla—From a shrub. (–)

Canola oil—Also known as rapeseed oil. (–)

Caprylic acid (octanoic acid)—Prepared by oxidation of n-octanol or by fermentation and distillation of fatty acids from coconut oil. (–)

Caramel color—Prepared by the heat treatment of food-grade carbohydrates such as dextrose, invert sugar, lactose, malt syrup, molasses, starch hydrolysates, sucrose; can be artificial; most often made from liquid corn syrup. (C,M,W)

Carboxymethylcellulose—From wood pulp and cotton linters. (–)

Carnauba wax—From the Brazilian wax palm, *Copernicia cerifera*. (–)

Carob bean gum (locust bean gum)—From pods of the carob (locust) tree. (–)

Carrageenan—From seaweeds, especially *Chondrus crispus*. (–)

Casein—Major protein in milk. (M)

Catsup (ketchup)—May contain corn syrup and vinegar. (C,W)

Cellulose—Obtained commercially from cotton and wood pulp. (–)

Cerelose—From corn. (C)

Chewing gum base—A combination of latex or chicle, plasticizers, antioxidants, and other preservatives. (–)

Chocolate:

> **Milk chocolate**—Usually contains cocoa butter, chocolate liquor, sugar, and milk; can contain added emulsifiers such as lecithin. *Always read the label:* Some brands of chocolate candy, such as plain *M&Ms*, list *peanuts* as an ingredient.

> **Semisweet chocolate** (bittersweet chocolate)—Must contain a minimum of 35-percent chocolate liquor. Chocolate is permitted to contain: milk, milk solids, nuts, coffee, honey, malt, salt, spices, and flavors.

> **Sweet or dark chocolate**—Usually contains chocolate liquor, cocoa butter, and sugar. U.S. standards demand that sweet chocolate contain at least 15-percent chocolate liquor by weight, and must be sweetened with sucrose, dextrose, or corn syrup solids.

Citric acid—Prepared by *Aspergillus* fermentation of carbohydrates such as corn or sugar beet molasses, or derived from citrus fruit or pineapple. Because of its low cost, sugar beet molasses is the preferred source. May also be prepared by *Candida* strains on glucose, molasses, or hydrocarbons. Citric acid is used to provide tartness in carbonated beverages, to adjust the pH of jams and jellies, or it is used alone or in combination with erythorbic acid to help prolong the shelf life of frozen fish. (C)

Cocoa (cocoa powder)—Prepared from chocolate liquor after the cocoa butter is removed. (–)

Cocoa butter—Fat obtained from cocoa beans. (–)

Cocoa butter substitutes—Can be produced from soy, corn, palm kernel, or cottonseed oils. Used in chocolate-flavored products. (C,S)

Cocoa, Dutched—Treated with an alkali such as sodium or potassium bicarbonate, to increase the pH of cocoa from its natural range of 5.4 to 5.8 to as high as 8.5. (–)

Coconut—The fruit of the coconut palm; not usually considered a "nut." (–)

Colorants—Although all added colors are considered to be "artificial," some food colorants are derived from "natural" sources and are exempt from FDA certification: annatto extract; dehydrated beets (beet powder); caramel; beta-carotene; cochineal; toasted cottonseed flour; ferrous gluconate (for ripe olives only); grape skin extract (enocianina); fruit and vegetable juice; carrot oil; paprika and paprika oleoresin; riboflavin; saffron; titanium dioxide; turmeric and turmeric oleoresin. (–)

In all, 33 colors are permitted for use in food. The two most widely used colors are Red No. 40 and FD&C Yellow No. 5 (tartrazine). General terms such as *artificial color* may appear on the label, except if a food contains tartrazine. Because it has been estimated that some 50,000 to 90,000 Americans are allergic to tartrazine, this coloring must be clearly identified on the label.

Conalbumen—From egg. (E)

Confectioners' glaze—Beeswax or carnauba wax, or shellac; used to polish candy. (–)

Confectioners' sugar—Usually mixed with cornstarch to prevent clumping. (C)

Cornstarch—From corn. (C)

Corn syrup—Prepared from cornstarch; contains glucose combined with dextrin and maltose. (C)

Cream of tartar (potassium bitartrate, potassium acid tartrate) —by-product of wine manufacture. (–)

Curcumin—Food color extracted from tumeric. (–)

Dextrin (starch gum)—A thickening agent formed by the hydrolysis of starch; produced from cornstarch, wheat, rice, potatoes, millet, or other cereals. (C,W)

Dextrose (corn sugar, glucose, dextroglucose, grape sugar)—Corn sugar commonly derived from cornstarch. (C)

Diacetyl—Used to impart a "buttery" flavor; synthesized from methyl ethyl ketone; used in butter starter distillates. (–)

Dicalcium diphosphate (monetite)—Mineral/synthetic. (–)

Diglycerides—Common emulsifiers derived primarily from vegetable oils. (C,P,S)

Disodium guanylate—Can be derived from soy or prepared from yeast. (S)

Disodium inosinate.—Salt of inosinic acid; can be prepared from soy or yeast. (S)

Disodium phosphate—Synthetic. (–)

EDTA—See Calcium disodium EDTA.

Edible bone phosphate—Steam-extract of animal bones. (–)

Egg albumin—Water-soluble proteins found in egg white. (E)

Emulsifier—General term for substances such as lecithin or mono- and diglycerides. (C,E,P,S)

Erythorbic acid—A source of modified food starch; derived from corn flour. (C)

Ester gum—From pine tree rosin and glycerol. (C,P,S)

Ethanol—See Ethyl alcohol.

Ethyl alcohol (ethanol)—May be synthesized or obtained by fermentation of sugars and starches. Any carbohydrate is a potential source of ethyl alcohol, but for beverage purposes cereal grains are the usual choice. (C,W)

Ethyl maltol—From maltol. (C,W)

Ethyl vanillin—Can be derived from *Sassafras officinale*. (–)

FD&C colors—Synthetic colors certified by the FDA for use in food and drugs.

Fatty acids—Most fatty acids, such as capric, caprylic, lauric, myristic, oleic, palmitic, or stearic acids, are derived from processing such edible fat sources as coconut, soybean, cottonseed, corn, and other vegetable oils. (C,P,S)

Fatty alcohols—Can be made from any fatty triglyceride or fatty acid, but primarily coconut, palm kernel, lard, tallow, and palm oil; and, sometimes, soybean, rapeseed, and fish oils are used. (S)

Flavors, artificial—May be a combination of natural and synthetic substances; for that reason anyone allergic to foods such as butter or nuts, for example, should avoid similarly named artificial flavorings.

Flour—(W)

Food shellac—Used as a glazing agent; four commercial grades are produced by various chemical processes. (–)

Food starch—May be derived from wheat, corn, sorghum, arrowroot, tapioca, or potatoes. (C,W)

Food starch, modified—See Modified food starch.

Fructose—Can be derived from the dahlia, Jerusalem artichoke, or other tubers; or by enzymic or microbial action on cornstarch. (C)

Furcellan gum—Extracted from *Furcellaria fastigiata*. (–)

Fumaric acid—Can be prepared by the fermentation of glucose with *Rhizopus*; or produced as a by-product of maleic anhydride production from benzene. (C)

Galactose—A monosaccharide occurring in milk sugar or lactose. (M)

Gelatin—Obtained by the partial hydrolysis of collagen—the chief component of animal skins, bones, and hide. (–)

Gluconic acid (dextronic acid, maltonic acid, glycogenic acid) —Prepared by the oxidation of glucose. (C)

Glucono delta-lactone—Prepared by the oxidation of glucose; contains gluconic acid. (C)

Glucose (dextrose, grape sugar)—A mixture of dextrose, maltose, and dextrin; derived from the hydrolysis of cornstarch. (C)

Glucose syrups (corn syrup, cornstarch, hydrolysate, starch syrup, confectioners' glucose, uncrystallizable syrup)—Prepared by the hydrolysis of maize or potato starches. (C)

Glutamates (glutamic acid, L-glutamic acid, MSG)—Prepared commercially by fermentation of a carbohydrate solution. (C,S,W)

Gluten—Found in wheat, rye, oats, barley, malt, and grain extracts and, possibly, buckwheat. (W)

Gluten-free grains, flours, and starches—Include corn, rice, millet, soybean, chickpea, and potato.

Glycerides—Common emulsifiers derived primarily from vegetable oils. (C,P,S)

Glycerin—See Glycerol.

Glycerol (glycerin)—A polyhydric alcohol recovered from the fractionation of fats and oils; often a product of soybean processing. (C,P,S)

Glyceryl abietate (glycerol ester of wood rosin)—From pine tree rosin and glycerol. (C,P,S)

Glyceryl monostearate (mono- and diglycerides of fatty acids) —Derived from fats; prepared from glycerin and fatty acids. (C,M,P,S)

Glycine—Amino acetic acid. (–)

Glycyrrhizic acid—Extracted from licorice. (–)

Guanine—Obtained from fish scales. (–)

Guar gum—From *Cyamopsis tetragonolobus.* (–)

Gum arabic—From *Acacia senegal.* (–)

Gum ghatti—From *Anogeissus latifolia.* (–)

Gum karaya—From *Stericulia urens.* (–)

Gum larch—From *Larix occidentalia.* (–)

Gum tragacanth—From *Astragalus gummifer.* (–)

High fructose corn syrup—A corn sweetener. (C)

Hydrochloric acid—Synthetic. (–)

Hydrogenated vegetable shortening—Any vegetable oil to which hydrogen is added. (C,P,S)

Hydrol (corn sugar molasses)—A by-product of crystallized dextrose. (C)

Hydrolyzed vegetable protein (HVP; also HPP, hydrolyzed plant protein)—Processed from vegetable proteins, such as corn, soybean, or wheat, which are hydrolyzed with an acid. (*Note:* Peanuts typically are not used to manufacture HVP in the United States; however some imported foods *might* contain HVP derived from peanuts.) (C,S,W)

Inosine 5'-disodium phosphate (Sodium 5'-inosinate)—can be produced from meat extract and sardines. (–)

Inosinic acid—From meat extract and sardines. (–)

Invert sugar—Invert sugar syrup can be produced by adding sodium bicarbonate and an inverting acid, such as tartaric or hydrochloric, to granulated sugar. (–)

Invertase—Enzyme from yeast. (–)

Iodized Salt—Often contains dextrose. (C)

Isomerose (high fructose corn syrup)—From corn. (C)

Japan wax (Japan tallow, vegetable wax)—From a tree fruit. (–)

Kaolin—Mineral found in granite. (–)
Karaya gum—Exudate of the *Sterculia urens* tree. (–)

Lactalbumin—Derived from whey. (M)
Lactic acid—Produced by milk-souring organisms; can be manufactured by the fermentation of cabohydrates (glucose, sucrose, or lactose) with *Bacillus acidilactic;* a by-product of
corn processing produced by the controlled fermentation of
highly refined sucrose, potato starch, molasses, corn sugar,
or milk whey. (C,M)
Lactic culture—See Lactic fermenting agents.
Lactic fermenting agents—Lactobacilli are used to ferment cabbage to sauerkraut and to prepare some types of pickles and
olives; may be cultured on milk. (M)
Lactose—Produced from whey; can be hydrolyzed into glucose
and galactose; can be fermented into lactic acid and butyric
acid. (M)
Lactylated fatty acid esters of glycerol and propane-1,2-diol—
Prepared from lactic acid. (C,M)
Lactylic esters of fatty acids—Prepared from lactic acid and fatty
acids. (C,M)
Lard—From hogs. (–)
Lecithin—A fatty substance consisting of glycerol, fatty acids,
phosphoric acid, and choline. Pure lecithin, a phosphatide,
accounts for only about 15 percent of commercial lecithin
products, which are usually 30-percent fatty oil. Most commercial lecithin is derived from soybeans; however, if it is
not qualified as soya lecithin on the label, it might have been
derived from other vegetable oils, including corn, rapeseed,
peanut, sunflower or safflower, or it could have been derived
from eggs; however, egg lecithin is of little commercial importance in U.S. food production. (C,E,P,S)
Levulose (fructose)—From corn. (C)
Lipoxidase—Enzymes obtained from soybean processing. (S)
Livetin—From eggs. (E)
Locust bean gum (carob bean gum)—From fruit of the carob tree
Ceratonia siliqua. (–)

Magnesium carbonate—Naturally occurring. (–)
Magnesium oxide—Mineral. (–)

Magnesium hydroxide (periclase)—Mineral. (–)

Magnesium phosphate (newberyite)—Mineral. (–)

Magnesium sulphate (Epsom salts)—From the sea. (–)

Malic acid—Prepared by the hydration of fumaric acid or maleic acid. (C)

Malt—Usually germinated barley; can also be made from yeast-fermented corn, wheat, or rice. (C,W)

Malted milk—Powder made of dried milk, malted barley, and wheat flour. (M,W)

Malt flavoring—May be derived from corn or wheat. (C,W)

Malt syrup—(C,W)

Maltodextrin—Prepared by partial hydrolysis of cornstarch with acids and enzymes; or can be produced from barley starch in the manufacture of malt. (C,W)

Maltol—From roasted malt or tree bark; can be obtained by alkaline hydrolysis of streptomycin salts. (C,W)

Maltose (malt sugar)—A product of sprouted grain, maltose can be produced commercially by the hydrolysis of starch (from soybeans, rice, millet, cereal, or potatoes) with yeast or an enzyme, such as beta-amylase. It is an intermediate formed in brewing, distilling, and vinegar manufacture. (C,S,W)

Mannitol—Synthesized from sugar or corn. (C)

Methyl glucoside—From corn. (C)

Microcrystalline wax—Prepared from petroleum. (–)

Miso—Product of soybean fermentation. (S)

Modified cornstarch—From corn. (C)

Modified food starch—Starch derived from cereal grains and potatoes that is treated with chemicals such as vinyl acetate, acetic anyhdride, or succinic anhydride; often derived from corn or wheat. (C,W)

Modified starch—see Modified food starch.

Modified tapioca starch—Prepared from the root of the cassava plant. (–)

Modified vegetable protein—May be derived from soybean, corn, or wheat. In Europe, peanut is also a common source. (C,S,W) (C,P,S,W for imported foods)

Molasses—Derived from sugarcane; some manufacturers use sulfur dioxide in the clarifying process. (–)

Monoglyceride citrate—Mixture of glyceryl monooleate and its citric acid monoester (contains 14 to 17 percent citric acid). (C)

Mono- and diglycerides—Emulsifiers derived primarily from vegetable oils; often derived from soy, corn, cottonseed, or palm oils; prepared by treating fat or oil with glycerine. (C,P,S)

Monocalcium phosphate—Derived by neutralizing phosphoric acid with lime at high temperatures. (–)

Monoglycerides, edible vegetable—See Mono- and Diglycerides.

Monosodium glutamate (MSG)—Wheat gluten was originally used as a raw material when industrial production of MSG began in 1909; beet sugar waste was also used in the past, but today most commercial MSG is produced by a fermentation process with *Micrococcus glutamicus* on acetic acid, or any common carbohydrate, such as soybean, seaweed, wheat, corn, or sugar beets. Penicillin is sometimes added during production to retard growth of unwanted microorganisms. (C,S,W)

Myristic acid—Long-chain fatty acid obtained from coconut oil, nutmeg butter, butter, lard, and other fats. (M)

Natto—Product of soybean fermentation. (S)

Nuts—General term for "tree nuts," which includes filberts, hazelnuts, cashews, pistachios, almonds, walnuts, butternuts, hickory nuts, pecans, Brazil nuts, chestnuts, pignolia, and macadamias, but not peanuts or coconuts. (N)

Oleoresin—This term is often used with spices, such as oleoresin of paprika; it indicates that the essential oil and resin has been extracted from a substance by using alcohol, ether, or acetone. (–)

Ovalbumin—From egg. (E)

Ovomucin—From egg. (E)

Ovomucoid—From egg. (E)

Palm kernel oil—Obtained by squeezing boiled fruit of the oil palm. (–)

Palmitic acid—Obtained from palm oil, Japan wax, or Chinese vegetable tallow. (–)

Palm oil—Obtained by boiling fruit of the oil palm. (–)

Papain—From unripe papaya. (–)

Peanuts—Botanically related to peas, peanuts are legumes, not true nuts. (P)

Pectins—Produced commercially from fruit peel and pulp. (–)

Penicillium—Organisms responsible for ripening of Camembert and Roquefort cheeses.

Peptones—Produced by partial hydrolysis of casein, soy, egg, whey. (E,M,S)

Phosphoric acid—Prepared by the action of sulfuric acid on tricalcium phosphate. (–)

Phosvitin—From egg. (E)

Polydextrose—Made from a mixture of glucose, sorbitol, and citric acid. (C)

Polyglycerol esters of fatty acids—Can be manufactured from corn, cottonseed, palm, peanut, safflower, sesame, or soybean oils, or from lard or tallow. (C,P,S)

Polyglycerol polyricinoleate—From castor oil. (–)

Polysorbates (Polysorbate 60, 65, 80)—See Sorbitans.

Potassium acid tartrate—By-product of wine manufacture. (–)

Potassium bicarbonate—Synthetically derived. (–)

Potassium bisulfite—Sulfiting agent. (–)

Potassium bromate—Synthetic bleaching agent for flour. (–)

Potassium gluconate—Salt of gluconic acid. (C)

Potassium hydroxide—Synthetic. (–)

Potassium metabisulfite—Sulfiting agent. (–)

Potassium nitrate—Naturally occurring. (–)

Potassium nitrite—Naturally occurring. (–)

Potassium sorbate—Prepared from sorbic acid and potassium hydroxide. (–)

Potassium sulphate—Naturally occurring. (–)

Propionic acid—A fatty-acid prepared by chemical synthesis or bacterial fermentation; can be derived from natural gas, wood pulp, or petroleum. (–)

Propyl gallate—Synthetic antioxidant. (–)

Propylene glycol—Alcohol derived from petroleum; used in antifreeze solutions and as a solvent. (–)

Propylene glycol monostearate—Produced from propylene glycol and a hydrogenated vegetable oil. (C,P,S)

Quercitol (acorn sugar)—From acorns. (N)

Quinine—Alkaloid extracted from *Cinchona* tree bark. (–)

Refiners syrup—From raw sugar. (–)

Rennet—A preparation from the lining of a calf's stomach. (–)
Resinous glaze—See Confectioners' glaze.
Riboflavin—Vitamin B$_2$. (–)
Roquefort cheese—Ripened by species of *Penicillium*. (M)

Saccharin—Noncaloric, artificial sweetener. (–)
Salt—May contain dextrose as a stabilizer, if iodized. (–)
Shellac (confectioners' glaze)—Refined, bleached resin secreted by the insect, *Kerria lacca*. (–)
Silicon dioxide—Mineral. (–)
Simethicone—From dimethylpolysiloxane and silica gel or silicone dioxide. (–)
Smoke flavoring—Extract of hickory or maple wood smoke. (–)
Sodium acid pyrophosphate—Often used as an ingredient in baking powder. (–)
Sodium aluminum phosphate—Synthetic. (–)
Sodium benzoate—Salt of benzoic acid. (–)
Sodium bicarbonate—Derived from the burning of limestone. (–)
Sodium bisulfite—Sulfiting agent. (–)
Sodium chloride—Table salt. (–)
Sodium choleate—Ox bile extract. (–)
Sodium citrate—Salt of citric acid. (C)
Sodium erythrobate—May be derived from corn. (C)
Sodium gluconate—Salt of gluconic acid. (C)
Sodium guanylate—Prepared synthetically; or isolated from sardines or yeast. (–)
Sodium lactate—Salt of lactic acid. (C,M)
Sodium metabisulfite—Sulfiting agent. (–)
Sodium nitrate—Naturally occurring. (–)
Sodium nitrate—Derived from sodium nitrate by chemical or bacterial action. (–)
Sodium phosphate—Salt of phosphoric acid. (–)
Sodium 5'-ribonucleotide—Mixture of disodium guanylate and disodium inosinate (should be avoided by those with gout or on a purine-restricted diet.) (S)
Sodium sesquicarbonate (trona)—From saline residues. (–)
Sodium stearoyl-2-lactylate—From lactic acid and stearic acid. (C,M,P,S)
Sodium sulfite—Sulfiting agent. (–)
Sodium sulphate (henardite, mirabilite)—Naturally occurring. (–)

Sorbase—Fermented from sorbitol. (C)

Sorbic acid—Obtained from the fruits of the mountain ash or synthesized. (–)

Sorbitans (including Span 20, 65, 80)—Derived from sorbitol and fatty acids. (C,P,S)

Sorbitol—From corn. (C)

Soy sauce (soya sauce)—From fermented soybeans, often with added wheat. (S,W)

Soya lecithin—From soy. (S)

Soya protein—From soy. (S)

Soybean oil—From soy. (S)

Stannous chloride—Produced by the action of hydrochloric acid on tin. (–)

Starch—Corn and tapioca are the major commercial sources; however, starch can be extracted from any cereal grain or tuber. (C,W)

Starter cultures—May be prepared in milk. (M)

Starter distillate (butter starter distillate)—Bacteria grown on skim milk fortified with citric acid. (M,C)

Stearic acid—Prepared by the hydrogenation of cottonseed and other vegetable oils or from edible tallow. (C,P,S)

Stearyl tartrate—From tartaric acid. (–)

Succinic acid—Hydrogenation of maleic or fumaric acid. (C)

Sucrose—Obtained from sugarcane and sugar beets. (–)

Sugar (cane sugar, liquid sugar)—From sugarcane and sugar beets. (–)

Sucrose fatty acid esters—Derived from sucrose and edible tallow. (–)

Sulfuric acid (oil of vitriol)—From sulphur dioxide. (–)

Table salt—Most table salt is plain, noniodized sodium chloride without any additives. In Japan, however, some table salt is coated with up to 10-percent MSG.

Talc—Mineral. (–)

Tannic acid—Solvent extraction of nut galls of *Quercus* (oak).

Tapioca flour—Food starch from the root of the cassava. (–)

Tartaric acid—By-product of wine manufacture. (–)

TBHQ (tert-butylhydroquinone)—Synthetic antioxidant. (–)

Tempeh—From soy fermentation. (S)

Textured vegetable protein—See Hydrolyzed vegetable protein.

Thiamine mononitrate—Vitamin B_1. (–)

Titanium dioxide—Naturally-occurring white pigment. (–)

Tocopherol (alpha-tocopherol)—Steam distillation of edible vegetable oil products. (C,P,S,W)

Tofu—A soybean product with added gypsum. (S)

Urease—Enzyme from soybean processing. (S)

Vanilla extract—Most commercial extracts contain alcohol; some brands also have added corn syrup. (C,W)

Vanillin (Ethyl vanilllin)—Can be prepared from eugenol (oil of cloves), guaiacol, and lignin (a product of paper manufacture). (–)

Vegetable gums—Can include locust bean, gum arabic or acacia, gum tragacanth or guar gum (–), or xanthan gum, which is a product of corn sugar fermentation. (C)

Vegetable lecithin—From corn, peanut, or soy. (C,P,S)

Vegetable oil—General term that can indicate oil obtained from any tree crop or seed, including soybean; sunflower; palm, palm kernel, and coconut; rapeseed; cottonseed; peanut; olive; sesame; corn and safflower. (C,P,S)

Vegetable protein (textured vegetable protein)—See Hydrolyzed vegetable protein.

Vinegar—Five types of vinegars are typically used in the United States: distilled white (produced by natural fermentation of grain or alcohol); apple cider (fermented from apple juice); corn or maize sugar vinegar (from corn sugar); wine vinegar (from red wines); malt vinegar (from malt or barley). (C,W)

Vitamin A—Extracted from fish-liver oils. (–)

Vitamin B (B_1, B_2, B complex)—Produced synthetically or derived from yeast or rice. (–)

Vitamin C (ascorbic acid, calcium ascorbate, sodium ascorbate) —Large-scale production involves use of *Acetobacter suboxidans* fermentation of calcium d-gluconate or the oxidation of l-sorbose. (C)

Vitamin D (D_2)—Produced by UV irradiation of sterols obtained from yeast or fish-liver oil. (–)

Vitamin E—From soybean processing; can be derived from wheat germ oil. (S,W)

Vitellin—From egg. (E)

Whey—Derived from milk. (M)

Whey solids—Dried whey solids are nearly 75 percent lactose. (M)

Xanthan gum—Produced by the microorganism *Xanthomonas campestris*, which is grown commercially on a medium of glucose (corn syrup). (C)

Xylitol—Carbohydrate alcohol used as a synthetic sweetener; commercial production from birch tree chips, beech, hardwoods, almond and pecan shells, cornstalks, and cobs heated with sulfuric acid.

Yeast (Baker's, Brewer's, Torula, dried or smoked)—A fungus often grown on a carbohydrate base. (–)

Yeast nutrients—Yeast food nutrients may contribute miniscule amounts of carbohydrate to a food product; malt is a typical nutrient media for yeast. (C,W)

Zein—From corn; used as a binder in tablet making and as a protective coating on confections. (C)

Food Products Containing Tartrazine (FD&C Yellow No. 5)

ALBA '77, FIT'N FROSTY:
  Vanilla
BANANA CREAM PIE MIX:
  (Concord)
BUTTERSCOTCH MORSELS:
  (Nestlé)
CAKE MIX:
  (Duncan Hines):
    Butter Recipe Fudge
    Butter Recipe Golden
    Deluxe Carrot
    Deluxe Devil's Food
    Deluxe Yellow
  (Sweet 'n Low):
    Lemon
    Yellow
CAKE- AND CANDY-MAKING INGREDIENTS:
  Cake Mate Glossy Red Decorating Gel
  (Wilton):
    Candy Color:
      Orange
      Red
      Yellow
    Candy Melts, chocolate
    Center Mix, lemon
CANDY:
  (Andes):

    Creme de Menthe
    Mint Parfait
Bingo Caramels & Taffy Squares
Bonkers:
    Chewy Chocolate
(Brach's):
    Circus Peanuts
    Conversation Hearts
    Dessert Mints
(Cadbury's):
    Mini Eggs
(Charles):
    Fruit Drops
    Root Beer Barrels
    Spearmint Drops
Chuckles:
    Fruit Jellies
    Jelly Candy
    Jelly Rings
    Spice Sticks & Drops
Dots
Fruit Choos
Fruit Slices (Maillard)
Good & Fruity
Good & Plenty
(Heide):
    Candy Corn with Honey
    Chocolate Babies
    Gummi Bears
    Jelly Eggs
    Jujyfruits
Jelly Beans:
    (Jelly Belly) Very Cherry
    (Rodda) Jelly Eggs
Jolly Rancher Candy Kisses
(Luden's):
    Honey-Lemon Cough Drops
    L's Jells
M&M's:
    Peanut
    Plain

Marshmallow:
  (Rhodda):
    Bunnies
    Cats
    Peeps
    Pumpkins
    Snowmen
    Trees
Menthos, mixed fruit
Mighty Bite:
  Apple
  Banana
Necco Wafers
Now & Later:
  Apple
  Banana
  Chocolate
  Mystery Mix
  Pineapple
  Rainbow
(Richardson) *After Dinner* Jelly Center Mints
Royals Mint Chocolates
(Russell Stover):
  Butterscotch Squares
  Fruit Jellies
  Honeysuckle Straws
  Lemon Squares
  Mint Squares
  Rosebud Mints
Skittles
Starburst
(Stark) Gummi Hearts of Gold
(Switzer Clark):
  Anise Mints
  Assorted Jelly Mints
  Butter Mints
  Pastel Mints
(Willy Wonka):
  DinaSour Eggs
  Everlasting Gobstopper

  Rinky Dinks
  Runts
  Tart 'n Tinys
CARAMEL APPLE WRAP (Concord)
CHEESECAKE MIX:
 (Jell-O)
COCKTAIL MIX:
 (Giroux):
  Daiquiri
  Margarita
  Sweet and Sour
  Tom Collins
COOKIES:
 (Duncan Hines):
  Butterscotch Chocolate Chip
 (Keebler):
  Fudge Sticks
 (Stella D'Oro):
  Anginetti
  Anisette Sponge
  Anisette Toast
  Breakfast Treats
  Lady Stella Assortment
COOKIES, mix:
 (Sweet 'n Low) Chocolate Chip
CUSTARD MIX:
 (Jell-O):
  Golden Egg
 (Sweet 'n Low):
  Chocolate
  Lemon
  Vanilla
DRINK MIXES:
 (Crystal Light):
  Caribbean Cooler
  Citrus Blend
  Iced Tea with Lemon
 (Fla-Vor-Aid):
  Sugar-Free Lemonade
  Unsweetened:
   Lemon-Lime

Orange
(Sweet 'n Low):
  Cherry
  Fruit Punch
FRENCH'S:
Food Colors:
  Egg Shade
  Green
  Yellow
Imitation Flavors and Extracts:
  Banana
  Butter
  Pineapple
  Pistachio
Seasoning Blends:
  Butter Salt
  Lemon & Parsley Salt
  Seasoning Salt
Cake Decorations:
  Coconut Flavors
  Confetti
  Flowers
  Gold Dragees
  Green Sugar
  Nonpareils
  Rainbow Mix
  Sequins
  Yellow Sugar
Lemon Pie Filling
Potato Products:
  Cheese Scalloped
  Tangy Au Gratin
Sauce Mixes:
  Potato Casserole Au Gratin
  Potato Casserole, Scalloped
FROSTING:
  (Duncan Hines) Vanilla
  (Pillsbury) Frosting Supreme, Vanilla
FROSTING MIX:
  (Sweet 'n Low) Chocolate

FROZEN CONFECTIONS:
  Life Savers Flavor Pops
  (Pop-Ice) Freezer Bars:
    Lemon-Lime
FRUIT DRINKS:
  (Flav-O-Rich) Lemon Lime
GATORADE:
  Lemon-Lime
GREEN GIANT:
  Baked Entrées:
    Boneless Beef Ribs in BBQ Sauce
    Chicken in BBQ Sauce
    Chicken in Herb & Butter Sauce
    Chicken Lasagna
    Enchilada Sonora Style
    Lasagna
    Spinach Lasagna
    Stuffed Cabbage
    Stuffed Peppers
    Swiss Steak with Gravy
  Boil-in-Bag Entrées:
    Beef Stew
    Lasagna
    Salisbury Steak
  Boil-in-Bag Vegetables, Valley Combination:
    American Style
    Italian Style
    Japanese Style
    Mexican Style
  Polybag Vegetables:
    Broccoli-Carrot Fanfare
    Corn-Broccoli Bounty
  Side Dishes:
    Jubilee Rice
    Rice 'n Broccoli in Cheese Sauce
    Stuffed Potatoes with Cheese-flavored Topping
    Stuffed Potatoes with Sour Cream and Chives
  Twin Pouch Boil-in-Bag Entrées:
    Beef Chow Mein
    Beef Burgundy

Beef Stroganoff
Cashew Chicken
Chicken à la King
Chicken & Noodles
Chicken Cacciatore
Chicken Chow Mein
Chicken Provencal
Chicken with Garden Vegetables
Salisbury Steak
Shrimp Creole
Shrimp Fried Rice
Shrimp in Creamy Herb Sauce
Spaghetti & Meatballs
Steak & Green Peppers
Sweet & Sour Chicken
Sweet & Sour Meatballs
Szechwan Beef
Turkey in Gravy
GRANOLA BARS:
 Kudos, Peanut Butter
ICE CREAM:
 (Welsh Farms):
  Mint Chocolate Chip
ICE CREAM CAKE ROLL (Green's)
LEMONADE, mix:
 (Sweet 'n Low)
LEMON COCKTAIL MIX, bottled:
 Mi-Lem' 3 'n 1
LIME JUICE:
 (Giroux), sweetened
MACARONI & CHEESE:
 (Golden Grain) Macaroni and Cheddar
MOUSSE MIX:
 (Jell-O):
  Chocolate Mousse Pie
  Rich & Lucious, Chocolate Fudge
(San Sucre):
  Cheesecake
  Lemon
PET:
 Deep Dish Pie Crust, Frozen

Pecan Twirls (Aunt Fanny's)
PILLSBURY:
   Apple Cinnamon Coffee Cake Mix
   Black Forest Ultimate Brownie Mix
   Bundt Cake Mixes—all flavors except: Tunnel of Fudge and
      Chocolate Mousse
   Cake & Cookie Decorator Icing:
      Green
      Yellow
   Chicken Gravy Mix
   Coconut Fudge Jumbles
   Cupcake Mixes, Pudding Pocket:
      Devils Food/Vanilla
      Yellow/Fudge
   Figurines—all flavors except: Chocolate-Caramel and Double
      Chocolate
   Frosting Mixes:
      Coconut Almond
      Coconut Pecan
   Hungry Jack Panshakes
   Hungry Jack Potato Flakes
   Instant Breakfast—all flavors except: Vanilla
   Milk Break Bars, Milk-flavor
   Pie Crust Mix and Sticks
   Pillsbury Plus Cake Mixes:
      Banana
      Butter Recipe
      Carrot 'n Spice
      Fudge Marble
      German Chocolate
      Lemon
      Strawberry
      Yellow
   Quick Bread Mix—all flavors except: Cherry Nut, Date, and
      Banana
   Ready-to-Spread Frosting Supreme:
      Caramel Pecan
      Chocolate Chip
      Coconut Almond
      Coconut Pecan

Cream Cheese
Lemon
Sour Cream Vanilla
Strawberry
Vanilla
Refrigerated Products:
　All Ready Pie Crust
　Artificial Butter Flavor Butter Biscuits
　Butterflake Dinner Rolls
　Cookies:
　　Oatmeal Raisin
　　Sugar
　Crescent Rolls
　Good 'n Buttery Big Country Biscuits
　Hungry Jack Butter Tastin' Flaky Biscuits
　Sweet Rolls—all varieties
　Turnovers—all flavors
　Rich 'N Easy Vanilla Frosting Mix
　Streusel Swirl Cake Mixes—all flavors
PLANTERS:
　Cheez Balls
POTATO CHIPS:
　Pringle's, Cheez-ums
PUDDING, MIX:
　(Jell-O):
　　Americana, Rice
　　Instant, Pistachio
　(My-T-Fine):
　　Chocolate
　　Vanilla
PUDDING POPS (Jell-O):
　Chocolate-Vanilla Swirl
　Vanilla
REESE'S PIECES (Hershey)
ROLLS:
　(Martin's) Potato
SALAD DRESSING:
　(Seven Seas) Green Goddess
　(Wish-Bone) Lite Italian

SHERBET:
  (Flav-O-Rich):
    Lime
    Rainbow
SHRIMP, frozen:
  (Carnation) Shrimp Crisps
SMUCKER'S:
  Butterscotch Topping
SNACKS, CHIPS, PUFFS:
  (Charles):
    Bacon 'N Cheddar Potato Chips
    Cheese Popcorn
    Cheese Twists
    Fried Twists
    Nacho Tostadas
  (Snyder's):
    Cheese Twists
  (Wise):
    Crunchy Cheez Doodles
    Nacho Cheese Bravos
SOFT DRINKS:
  Aunt Wicks Rootbeer
  Mountain Dew
  (Shasta) Citrus Mist
TONTINO'S:
  Classic Casseroles—all flavors
  Fox Deluxe Pizza—all varieties
  My Classic:
    Lasagna
    Pizza—all varieties
  Toaster Strudel—all flavors
  Tontino's Party, Extra! Pizza—all varieties
TWINKIES
WAFFLES, frozen:
  (Downyflake):
    Buttermilk
    Regular
  (Eggo) Homestyle

Clues to Foods and Recipes, or What's in a Name?

If you were allergic to eggs you would probably avoid egg foo young and egg drop soup in a Chinese restaurant, but should you also have to avoid egg rolls—those deep-fried, rolled-up wrappers of noodle dough that are filled with minced vegetables, meat, and shrimp? Interestingly, I noticed that most of the frozen egg rolls sold in my local supermarket did not contain eggs. Nor did some commercial brands of Caesar salad dressing, despite the fact that the classic recipe for Caesar salad always includes a coddled egg.

What this means to a food-sensitive individual is: Never judge a food by its name alone. There may not be any eggs in an egg roll, just as there aren't any eggs in an egg cream (a soda-fountain concoction of syrup, milk, and seltzer water), and an egg-sensitive individual could safely eat some brands of frozen egg rolls and some bottled Caesar dressings, but would be advised to avoid those same foods in a restaurant, unless the cook was consulted about the ingredients.

The surprise ingredient in egg rolls may not be eggs, but *peanut butter*. Dr. Stephen L. Taylor, an Associate Professor at the University of Wisconsin's Department of Food, Microbiology and Toxicology, says, "Some Oriental restaurants have a nasty habit of using peanut butter to glue down the ends of an eggroll so that when they put them in the fryer, they don't unroll."

Recipes, Main Dishes, and Foreign Foods that Could Be Dangerous to Your Health

You're allergic to eggs and your hostess has just announced that dinner will be an international delight: Greek avgolemono soup; Caesar salad; beef Wellington with Yorkshire pudding; asparagus with Hollandaise sauce and, for dessert, zabaglione. Sounds delicious; but all you'll be able to eat is the roast beef (if you peel away the pastry crust) and plain asparagus spears. Everything else, from the lemon-flavored soup to the Italian dessert, is loaded with eggs.

Instead of listing general categories of foods such as pies, pastries, and candies that should be avoided by those allergic to corn, milk, eggs, or nuts, I looked through several dozen cookbooks and encyclopedias for specific recipes or cooking terms that often contain unusual or unexpected ingredients. As an example: Most salads don't contain wheat, unless they're topped with croutons, but tabbouli, a Middle Eastern dish made from bulgur wheat, tomatoes, parsley, mint, lemon juice, and olive oil, is one exception that comes to mind.

The following list does not note all of the possible allergens a food might contain—there are too many cooks with too many variations to make that possible. However, it does list those allergens that are somewhat unusual and might catch you off guard.

RECIPES USUALLY PREPARED WITH CORN:

Anadama bread
Brunswick stew
Hominy
Hoppin' John
Hush puppies
Indian pudding
Johnnycake
Polenta
Scrapple
Spoon bread
Succotash
Tacos
Taffy
Tamales
Tortillas

RECIPES USUALLY PREPARED WITH EGGS:

Angel food cake
Avgolemono soup, sauce
Baked Alaska
Beárnaise sauce

Billi Bi soup
Brioche
Ceasar salad
Chocolate Mousse
Clarified bouillon, consomme
Cream puffs
Crepes suzette
Eclairs
Empanadas
Flan
Frangipane
French crullers
Fried rice
Fritata
Genoise
Gnocchi
Hollandaise sauce
Ladyfingers
Macaroons
Madeleines
Mandeltorte
Mayonnaise
Meringue pie
Mornay sauce
Mousseline sauce

Nesselrode pie
Newburg sauce
Nougat candy
Oeufs à la neige
Pavlova
Popovers
Pot de creme au chocolat
Quiche
Seven-minute frosting
Souffles
Spaetzle
Spaghetti carbonara
Sponge cake
Steak tartare
Syllabub
Tempura
Tom and Jerry cocktail
Tortes
Trifle
Vol-au-vent
Welsh rabbit/Rarebit
Yorkshire pudding
Zabaglione
Zeppole
Zuppa inglese

Also, any foods prepared *à la Russe, Divan or Polonaise*

RECIPES USUALLY PREPARED WITH MILK:

Bechamel sauce
Beárnaise sauce
Billi Bi soup
Bisque soups
Cream sauces
Cream soups
Frangipane
Gnocchi

Hollandaise sauce
Mornay sauce
Mousseline sauce
Newburg sauce
Tortoni
Trifle
Vichyssoise
White sauce

Also, foods prepared *a l'Allemande, a la Hongroise, a la maitre d'hotel, a la mode, alla milanese, amandine, au gratin, divan, smitane, Tetrazzini or Veronique*

RECIPES USUALLY PREPARED WITH NUTS:

Frangipane
German chocolate cake
Linzertorte
Mandeltorte
Marzipan
Mincemeat
Mont Blanc aux marrons
Also, any foods prepared *amandine*

Nougat candy
Pesto sauce
Pralines
Tortoni
Strudels
Waldorf salad

RECIPES USUALLY PREPARED WITH SHELLFISH:

Billi Bi soup
Bouillabaisse
Cacciucco
Chupe
Cioppino

Coquilles
Gumbo
Jambalaya
Paella
Peixada

RECIPES USUALLY PREPARED WITH WHEAT:

Bechamel sauce
Bisque soups
Cream sauces
Cream soups
Drawn butter
Empanadas
Frangipane
Gefilte fish
Gnocchi

Mornay sauce
Schnitzel
Tabbouli salad
Teriyaki
Tortes
Tortillas, wheat
Trifle
White sauce

Also, foods prepared *a l'Allemande, a la Hongroise, au gratin, Tetrazzini* or *Veronique*

E Numbers: Deciphering Labels on Imported Foods

You've just picked up an exquisite box of imported cookies, and you'd like to know if tartrazine (FD&C Yellow No. 5) or any sulfiting agents were used as ingredients. The label states that the cookies contain food colors and preservatives, but instead of specific chemical names, there are only numbers. Welcome to the European Economic Community (EEC), where "E Numbers" have replaced names on package labels.

To facilitate the movement of food products within the EEC, or Common Market, a list of additives "generally recognized as safe" was generated and each was assigned a code. Instead of encumbering the label with lengthy words such as mono- and diglycerides of fatty acids or sodium stearoyl-2-lactylate, the label simply states: Emulsifiers (E 471, E 481).

If you want to avoid certain food colors, such as tartrazine (E 102): or preservatives, such as sulfur dioxide (E 220), consult the following list of "E" Numbers before you purchase any imported foods:

PERMITTED COLORS (E 100–E 163)

E 100	Curcumin (an extract of turmeric)
E 101	Riboflavin, vitamin B_2
E 102	Tartrazine
E 103	Chrysoine
E 104	Quinoline yellow
E 105	Fast yellow
E 110	Orange yellows
E 111	Orange GGN
E 120	Cochineal

E 121	Orchil, orcein
E 122	Azorubine
E 123	Amaranth
E 124	Ponceau 4R
E 125	Scarlet GN
E 126	Ponceau 6R
E 127	Erythrosine
E 130	Anthraquinone blue
E 131	Patent blue V
E 132	Indigo carmine
E 140	Chlorophyll
E 141	Copper complexes of chlorophyll
E 142	Acid brilliant green BS
E 150	Caramel
E 151	Brilliant black BN
E 152	Black 7984
E 153	Carbon black
E 160	Carotenoids, including annatto, capsathin
E 161	Xanthophylls
E 162	Beetroot red
E 163	Anthocyanins
E 170	Calcium carbonate
E 171	Titanium dioxide
E 172	Iron oxides and hydroxides
E 173	Aluminum
E 174	Silver
E 175	Gold
E 180	Lithol-rubin BK
E 181	Burnt umber

PRESERVATIVES (E 200–E 299)

E 200	Sorbic acid
E 201	Sodium sorbate
E 202	Potassium sorbate
E 203	Calcium sorbate
E 210	Benzoic acid
E 211	Sodium benzoate
E 212	Potassium benzoate
E 213	Calcium benzoate
E 214	Ethyl p-hydroxybenzoate
E 215	Sodium p-hydroxybenzoate

E 216	Propyl p-hydroxybenzoate
E 217	Sodium p-hydroxybenzoate
E 218	Methyl p-hydroxybenzoate
E 220	Sulphur dioxide
E 221	Sodium sulfite
E 222	Acid sodium sulfite
E 223	Sodium metabisulfite
E 224	Potassium metabisulfite
E 226	Calcium sulfite
E 227	Calcium hydrogen sulfite
E 230	Biphenyl
E 231	Orthophenylphenol
E 232	Sodium orthophenylphenate
E 233	Thiabendazole
E 236	Formic acid
E 237	Sodium formate
E 238	Calcium formate
E 239	Hexamine
E 240	Boric acid
E 241	Borax (sodium tetraborate)
E 249	Potassium nitrite
E 250	Sodium nitrite
E 251	Sodium nitrate
E 252	Potassium nitrate
E 260	Acetic acid
E 261	Potassium acetate
E 262	Sodium diacetate
E 263	Calcium acetate
E 270	Lactic acid
E 280	Propionic acid
E 281	Sodium propionate
E 282	Calcium propionate
E 283	Potassium pripionate
E 290	Carbon dioxide

ANTIOXIDANTS (E 300–E 399)

E 300	Ascorbic acid
E 301	Sodium ascorbate
E 302	Calcium ascorbate
E 303	Ascorbyl diacetate
E 304	Ascorbyl palmitate
E 306	Tocopherols of natural origin; vitamin E

E 307	Alpha-tocopherol, synthetic
E 308	Gamma-tocopherol, synthetic
E 309	Delta-tocopherol, synthetic
E 310	Propyl gallate
E 311	Octyl gallate
E 312	Dodecyl gallate
E 320	BHA—Butylated hydroxyanisole
E 321	BHT—Butylated hydroxytoluene
E 322	Lecithins
E 325	Sodium lactate
E 326	Potassium lactate
E 327	Calcium lactate
E 330	Citric acid
E 331	Sodium citrate
E 332	Potassium citrate
E 333	Calcium citrate
E 334	Tartaric acid
E 335	Sodium tartrate
E 336	Cream of tartar (potassium tartrate)
E 337	Sodium potassium tartrate
E 338	Phosphoric acid
E 339	Sodium orthophosphates
E 340	Potassium dihydrogen orthophosphates
E 341	Calcium phosphates

EMULSIFIERS, STABILIZERS, & THICKENERS (E 400–E 499)

E 400	Alginic acid
E 401	Sodium alginate
E 402	Potassium alginate
E 403	Ammonium alginate
E 404	Calcium alginate
E 405	1,2-propylene glycol alginate
E 406	Agar
E 407	Carrageenan
E 408	Furcelleran
E 410	Locust bean gum
E 411	Tamarind seed flour
E 412	Guar gum
E 413	Gum tragacanth
E 414	Gum arabic
E 415	Xanthan gum

E 420	Sorbitol
E 421	Mannitol
E 422	Glycerol
E 440	Pectins
E 450	Sodium and potassium polyphosphates
E 460	Microcrystalline cellulose
E 461	Methylcellulose
E 462	Ethylcellulose
E 463	Hydroxypropylcellulose
E 464	Hydroxyproylmethylcellulose
E 465	Methylethylcellulose
E 466	Carboxymethylcellulose
E 470	Sodium, potassium, and calcium salts of fatty acids
E 471	Mono- and diglycerides of fatty acids
E 472	Acetic, lactic, citric, and tartaric acid esters of mono- and diglycerides
E 473	Sucrose esters of fatty acids
E 474	Sucroglycerides
E 475	Polyglycol esters of fatty acids
E 477	Propylene glycol esters of fatty acids
E 480	Stearoyl-2-lactylic acid
E 481	Sodium stearoyl-2-lactylate
E 482	Calcium stearoyl-2-lactylate
E 483	Stearyl tartrate

MODIFIED STARCHES

E 1400	Dextrins
E 1401	Acid-treated starches
E 1402	Alkaline-treated starches
E 1403	Bleached starches

ADDITIVES UNDER CONSIDERATION FOR "E" PREFIXES

107	Yellow 2G
128	Red 2G
133	Brilliant blue FCF
154	Brown FK
155	Brown HT
296	Malic acid
297	Fumaric acid
350	Sodium malate
351	Potassium malate

352	Calcium malate
353	Metatartaric acid
355	Adipic acid
363	Succinic acid
370	1,4-Heptonolactone
375	Niacin
380	Ammonium citrates
385	Calcium disodium EDTA
416	Karaya gum
430	Polyoxyethylene (8) stearate
431	Polyoxyethylene stearate
432	Polysorbate 20
433	Polysorbate 80
434	Polysorbate 40
435	Polysorbate 60
436	Polysorbate 65
442	Ammonium phosphatides
476	Polyglycerol polyricinoleate
478	Lactylated fatty acid esters of glycerol
491	Sorbitan monostearate
492	Sorbitan tristearate
493	Sorbitan monolaurate
494	Sorbitan mono-oleate
495	Sorbitan monopalmitate
500	Sodium carbonates
501	Potassium carbonates
503	Ammonium carbonates
504	Magnesium carbonate
507	Hydrocholoric acid
508	Potassium chloride
509	Calcium chloride
510	Ammonium chloride
513	Sulfuric acid
514	Sodium sulfate
515	Potassium sulfate
516	Calcium sulfate
518	Magnesium sulfate
524	Sodium hydroxide
525	Potassium hydroxide
526	Calcium hydroxide
527	Ammonium hydroxide
528	Magnesium hydroxide

529	Calcium oxide
530	Magnesium oxide
535	Sodium ferrocyanide
536	Potassium ferrocyanide
540	Calcium phosphate dibasic
541	Sodium aluminum phosphates
542	Edible bone phosphate
544	Calcium polyphosphates
545	Ammonium polyphosphates
551	Silicon dioxide
552	Calcium silicate
553	Magnesium silicates; talc
554	Aluminum sodium silicate
556	Aluminum calcium silicate
558	Bentonite
559	Kaolin
570	Stearic acid
572	Magnesium stearate
575	Glucono delta-lactone
576	Sodium gluconate
577	Potassium gluconate
578	Calcium gluconate
620	L-glutamic acid
621	Monosodium glutamate
622	Monopotassium glutamate
623	Calcium glutamate
627	Sodium guanylate
631	Sodium 5-inosinate
635	Sodium 5-ribonucleotide
636	Maltol
637	Ethyl maltol
900	Simethicone
901	Beeswax
903	Carnauba wax
904	Shellac
905	Mineral hydrocarbons
907	Microcrystalline wax
920	L-cysteine hydrochlorides
924	Potassium bromate
925	Chlorine
926	Chlorine dioxide
927	Azodicarbonamide

References

Books

Asthma and Allergy Foundation of America. *The Allergy Encyclopedia*. New York: New American Library, 1981.

Benarde, M. A. *The Chemicals We Eat*. New York: American Heritage Press, 1971.

Bender, A. E. *Dictionary of Nutrition and Food Technology*. London: Butterworth, 1982.

Breneman, James C. (ed.) *Handbook of Food Allergies*. New York: Marcel Dekker, 1987.

Considine, D. M. and G. D. Considine (eds.) *Foods and Food Production Encyclopedia*. New York: Van Nostrand Reinhold, 1982.

Feingold, B. F. *Introduction to Clinical Allergy*. Springfield. Ill.: Thomas, 1973.

Furia, T. E. (ed.). *CRC Handbook of Food Additives*. Boca Raton, Fla.: CRC Press, 1980.

Kirk-Othmer Encyclopedia of Chemical Technology. New York: Wiley, 1980.

Leung, A. Y. *Encyclopedia of Common Natural Ingredients Used in Food, Drugs and Cosmetics*. New York: Wiley, 1980.

Marmion, D.M. *Handbook of U.S. Colorants for Foods, Drugs and Cosmetics*. New York: Wiley, 1979.

Office of the Federal Register. *Code of Federal Regulations*. Washington, D.C.: National Archives and Records Administration, 1986.

Pyke, M. *Food Science and Technology*. London: John Murray, 1981.

Tver, D. F. and P. Russell. *Nutrition and Health Encylopedia*. New York: Van Nostrand Reinhold, 1981.

Articles

American Academy of Allergy and Immunology Committee on Adverse Reactions to Foods. *Adverse Reactions to Foods*. U.S. Department of Health and Human Services, NIH Publication No. 84-2442, July 1984.

Bahna, S. L. "Control of Milk Allergy: A Challenge for Physicians, Mothers and Industry," *Annals of Allergy 41* (1):1–12, July 1978.

Bahna, S. L. and C. T. Furukawa. "Food Allergy: Diagnosis and Treatment," *Annals of Allergy 51* (6): 574–580, December 1983.

Bahna, S. L. and M. D. Gandhi. "Milk Hypersensitivity. I. Pathogenesis and Symptomatology," *Annals of Allergy 50* (4):218–223. April 1983.

———. "Milk Hypersensitivity. II. Practical Aspects of Diagnosis, Treatment and Prevention," *Annals of Allergy 50* (5):295–301. May 1983.

Bahna, S. L. and D. C. Heiner. "Serum IgE and IgD in Celiac Disease." *Clinical Research 25* (2):181, 1977.

Bentley, S. J., et al. "Food Hypersensitivity in Irritable Bowel Syndrome," *Lancet 2*, pp. 295–297, 1983.

Buckley, R. H. and D. Metcalfe. "Food Allergy," Journal American Medical Association *248* (20): 2627–2631, November 28, 1982.

Check, W. "Eat, Drink and Be Merry—or Argue about Food 'Allergy.' " *JAMA 250* (6):701–711, August 12, 1983.

"Death from Allergy to Food Spurs Study in Rhode Island," *New York Times*, July 7, 1986.

Dissanayake, A. S. "Jejunal Mucosal Recovery in Coeliac Disease in Relation to the Degree of Adherence to a Gluten-free Diet," *Quarterly Journal of Medicine 43* (170):161–185, April 1974.

Dissanayake, A. S., et al. "Lack of Harmful Effect of Oats on Small-intestinal Mucosa in Coeliac Disease," *British Medical Journal 4* (5938):189–191, 1974.

Harris, O. D. "Malignancy in Adult Coeliac Disease and Idiopathic Steatorrhoea," *American Journal of Medicine 42*:899–912, June 1967.

Herman, J. J., et al. "Allergic Reactions to Measles (Rubeola) Vaccine in Patients Hypersensitive to Egg Protein," *Journal of Pediatrics 102* (2):196–199, 1983.

Hughes, E. C. "Use of a Chemically Defined Diet in the Diagnosis of Food Sensitivities and the Determination of Offending Foods," *Annals of Allergy 40*, pp. 393–398, June 1978.

Institute of Food Technologists Panel on Food Safety and Nutrition. "Food Allergies and Sensitivities," *Food Technology*, September 1985, pp. 65–70.

Juhlin, L. "Incidence of Intolerance to Food Additives," *International Journal of Dermatology 19* (10):548–551, 1980.

Kuroume, T., et al. "Milk Sensitivity and Soybean Sensitivity in the Production of Eczematous Manifestations in Breast-fed Infants with Particular Reference to Intrauterine Sensitization," *Annals of Allergy 37*: 41–46, July 1976.

Lecos, C. "Food Preservatives: A Fresh Report," FDA Consumer, April 1984. pp. 23–25.

Lloyd-Still, J. D. "Chronic Diarrhea of Childhood and the Misuse of Elimination Diets," *Journal of Pediatrics 95* (1):10–13, July 1979.

———— "Where Have All the Celiacs Gone?" *Pediatrics 61*(6): 929–930, June 1978.

Lusas, E. W. "Food Uses of Peanut Proteins," Journal American Oil Chemists' Society *56*:425–430, 1979.

McCrae, W. Morrice, et al. "Neglected Coeliac Disease," *Lancet 1*:187–190, January 25, 1975.

"Milk Intolerance Tied to Normal Change in Digestion," *Modern Medicine*, October 1982, p. 41.

Miller, R. W. and C. Lecos. "Sweet Milk and Sour Stomachs," *FDA Consumer*, March 1984, p. 23.

Ormerod, A. D. and P. J. A. Holt. "Acute Utricaria Due to Alcohol," *Journal of Dermatology 108*, pp. 723–724, 1983.

Rainer, B., et al. "Allergenicity of Modified and Processed Foodstuffs," *Annals of Allergy 10*:675, 1952.

Saarinen, U. M. and M. Kajosaari. "Does Dietary Elimination in Infancy Prevent or Only Postpone a Food Allergy?" *Lancet. 1*, 166–167, January 26, 1980.

Soothill, J. F. "Some Intrinsic and Extrinsic Factors Predisposing to Allergy," *Proceedings Royal Society of Medicine 69*, 439–442, June 1976.

Speer, F. "Food Allergy: The Ten Common Offenders," *American Family Physician 13*(2):106–112, 1976.

Symposium Proceedings on Adverse Reactions to Foods and Food Additives. *The Journal of Allergy and Clinical Immunology 78* (1):125–252. July 1986.

Tattrie, N. H. and M. Yaguchi. "Protein Content of Various Processed Edible Oils," *Journal Institut Canadien de Science et Technologie 6* (4):289–290, 1973.

Taylor, S. L. "Peanut Oil Is Not Allergenic to Peanut-Sensitive Individuals," *Journal of Allergy and Clinical Immunology 68* (5):372–375, 1981.

Thompson, R. C. "Food Allergies: Separating Fact From 'Hype'," *FDA Consumer*, June 1986, pp. 25–27.

Wicher, K., et al. "Allergic Reactions to Penicillin Present in Milk," *JAMA. 208* (1):143–145, 1969.

Wicher, K. and R. E. Reisman. "Anaphylactic Reaction to Pencillin (or penicillin-like substance) in a Soft Drink," *Journal of Allergy and Clinical Immunology 66*(2):155–157, 1983.

Williams, C. "Intolerance to Additives," *Annals of Allergy 51*, 315–316, August 1983.

Unpublished Works:

Minutes of the August 20, 1986 Meeting of the Ad Hoc Advisory Committee on Hypersensitivity to Food Constitutents, Food and Drug Administration. (488 pp.)

Organizations and Sources of Information

Allergy Information Association
25 Poynter Drive, Room 7
Weston, Ontario, Canada M9R 1K8

American Academy of Allergy and Immunology
611 E. Wells Street
Milwaukee, Wisconsin 53202

American Digestive Disease Society
7720 Wisconsin Avenue
Bethesda, Maryland 20814

Asthma and Allergy Foundation of America
1302 18th Street NW
Washington, D.C. 20036

Feingold Association of the United States
P.O. Box 6550
Alexandria, Virginia 22306

National Dairy Council
6300 North River Road
Rosemont, Illinois 60018

National Institute of Allergy and Infectious Disease
9000 Rockville Pike
Bethesda, Maryland 20014

Specialty Manufacturers

Anglo-Dietetics Ltd.
P.O. Box 333
Wilton, Connecticut 06897

Bronson Pharmaceuticals
4526 Rinetti Lane
La Canada, California 91011

Ener-G Foods Inc.
P.O. Box 24723
Seattle, Washington 98124

Erewhon Natural Foods
236 Washington Street
Brookline, Massachusetts 02146

Lactaid, Inc.
P.O. Box 111
600 Fire Road
Pleasantville, N.J. 08232

Sandoz Nutrition
5320 W. 23 Street
Minneapolis, Minnesota 55440

Walnut Acres
Penns Creek, Pennsylvania 17862

Worthington Foods Inc.
900 Proprietors Road
Worthington, Ohio 43085